No More Snoring

A Proven Program for Conquering Snoring and Sleep Apnea

Victor Hoffstein, M.D.
Shirley Linde, Ph.D.

John Wiley & Sons, Inc.

New York • Chichester • Weinheim • Brisbane • Singapore • Toroi

Copyright © 1999 by Victor Hoffstein and Shirley Linde. All rights reserved

Published by John Wiley & Sons, Inc.

Published simultaneously in Canada

Library of Congress Cataloging-in-Publication Data

Hoffstein, Victor
   No more snoring : a proven program for conquering snoring and sleep apnea / Victor Hoffstein, Shirley Linde.
     p. cm.
   Includes index.
   ISBN 0-471-24375-2 (pbk. : alk. paper)
   1. Snoring—Treatment. 2. Sleep apnea—Treatment. 3. Insomnia—Treatment. 4. Sleep disorders—Treatment. I. Title.
RA786.3.H64 1999
616.8′498—dc21   98-16096

Printed in the United States of America

10 9 8 7 6 5 4 3 2 1

Contents

1

Many Snore, Few Are Treated

It is said that in 1843 John Wesley Hardin, the infamous Wild West gunfighter from Texas, shot and killed a loud snorer sleeping in the next room in a hotel in Abilene. He just couldn't put up with the noise any longer.

Things don't usually take such a violent turn, although many spouses have confessed to feeling almost as violent and frustrated after lying awake for hours, night after night, unable to sleep because of the loud repetitive rumbling erupting next to them again and again and again.

There are an estimated 88 million men and women in the United States who are snorers; some 40 million of them suffer on a regular, unrelenting, and usually nightly basis. Surveys indicate that 20 percent of the adult population snores, and some indicate that as many as 86 percent of men over 40 suffer from the problem. Specific numbers vary, but studies from all around the world show very large numbers of suffering snorers—and suffering snorers' partners.

In other words, there are hundreds of millions of snorers throughout the world, with the roar of snores rising to the skies from cities and villages all around the globe. Unfortunately, what most people don't realize is that snoring can be dangerous. And they also don't realize it can now be successfully treated.

Sleepless in Setauket

In a survey conducted by the Gallup Organization for the National Sleep Foundation in 1995 involving more than 1,000 adult men and women, more than half of the respondents had been told by others

1

that they snore, and one out of eight said they had been told that they also choke, gasp, or stop breathing for short times during sleeping. Statistics are similar in other countries.

Snorers and those who listen to them are sleepless in Seattle, Setauket, Seville, and São Paulo. In fact, in Setauket and more than a dozen other New York towns, a sleep researcher of New York University Medical Center distributed questionnaires to commuters at railroad stations. Of the 5,000 who answered the questionnaires, 40 percent said they were snorers, and 13 percent had the signs of sleep apnea, a more serious problem in which sleep is repeatedly interrupted with episodes of stopped breathing. Moreover, one out of four respondents said they had difficulty staying awake during the day while working, driving, or even talking on the phone. But few had ever received diagnosis or treatment. Most had never even asked for help. In fact, one National Family Opinion poll showed that only 4 percent of Americans have sought treatment for their snoring.

Not Just a Nuisance Condition

When most people think of snoring, they think of it as an almost humorous nuisance. But snoring can have very serious effects on the quality of your life and your health.

First, there are social ramifications. The social complications of snoring can be staggering. It can lead to social isolation, marital breakdowns, and chronic depression. It has threatened to break up couples on their honeymoon, gotten roommates kicked out, led to brawls in army barracks, kept potential relationships from progressing, and caused spouses to be banned to other rooms. In marriages all over the world, snoring is a nightly burden for both the snorer and the bedpartner. Wives and husbands—the silent suffering partners—lie awake next to their bedpartners every night, feeling angry and frustrated, building resentment, losing sleep. Others have moved to a different room to sleep. And some to different houses.

In addition, what most people don't know is that snoring can affect your quality of life in the daytime. Even though you may not realize it, snoring causes many brief arousals during your sleep that, when added up through the night, amount to enough lost sleep to affect how you feel and react the next day. Because of that, snoring can cause sleepiness at home, on the road, and on the job, and it can contribute to serious errors—sometimes catastrophic accidents. We'll tell you more of such incidents later—the facts are frightening.

Most people also don't realize that snoring can seriously affect your health, both on its own and because it often leads to episodes of gasping for air and stopped breathing called apnea. Sleep apnea can cause even more serious hazards to your health, and is sometimes even life-threatening. In some people these episodes of apnea can happen more than 100 times per hour.

Up until now the public—and even most physicians—have been unaware of just how hazardous to health snoring can be. Snorers seldom mention their problem to doctors and almost never seek medical help for it, and most physicians never even ask patients whether they snore. In fact, information about snoring and other sleep problems is seldom even taught in medical school or internship. A 1990 survey of U.S. medical schools showed little is taught to physicians about sleep in either the preclinical or clinical years.

But there has been a tremendous growth of knowledge at the research level, and treatments are now available. Unfortunately, many physicians in practice are still not receiving the information. Most members of the public and of the medical profession are unaware of the widespread impact of sleep disorders and the fact that treatments are available for them.

In fact, only recently have physicians and the public started to become aware of the extent to which snoring and other sleep disorders can lead to problems in people's lives. To assess how extensive the problem was, the U.S. Congress established a National Commission on Sleep Disorders Research. After studying the situation, the commission issued a report to Congress in 1992 called *Wake Up America* that labeled the low level of awareness of the impact of sleep disorders a national emergency. "The American public has been inappropriately denied the benefits of the research knowledge its tax dollars have supported," the commission reported. "This situation must be remedied without delay."

As a result, in 1993 the National Center on Sleep Disorders Research was established as part of the National Institutes of Health in the United States to deal with the many ramifications of sleep disorders and to educate physicians and the public about them. The commission urged physicians to discuss sleep problems with their patients.

In relation to apnea, the commission said the health costs for diagnosis and treatment of that alone might reach $60 billion. Dr. William Dement, head of the commission and professor of medicine at California's Stanford University, says, "Americans have gotten the message that good nutrition and plenty of exercise are important for health . . . but we haven't paid enough attention to the third pillar of good health, which is adequate sleep."

A typical study cited by the commission is one done in Finland by Dr. Kirsti Martikainen and other researchers who found habitual snoring, untreated, gets worse over time, often affecting daytime functioning more and more. Sleepiness was common in the Finnish men and women they studied, with 23 percent of the snorers reporting dozing off at the wheel because of sleepiness. But during the five years tracked by the investigators, none of the sufferers had sought or been given advice or treatment!

The evidence of just what snoring can do to your life and your health, only now becoming known, is startling.

The Hazards of Daytime Sleepiness

Snoring tonight can make both you and your bedpartner sleepy tomorrow. It can wake you up again and again throughout the night, making you and your nighttime partner sleepy the next day. The snorers, as well as their bedpartners, often stagger to work in the morning bleary-eyed and dragging from insufficient sleep. They may go through the day listless and irritable, inattentive, inefficient, feeling no joy from the day, only wanting to get through it.

Snoring interrupts sleep for brief periods, frequently even without the snorer's being aware of this. These interruptions show up as "blips" in brain activity in the sleep lab and are called "arousals." They cause what researchers call "fragmented sleep," which is not as restful. As a consequence, snorers frequently wake up not feeling refreshed, and throughout the day they continue to feel tired, sleepy, and fatigued.

Now research studies all over the world show that snorers also tend to have memory and concentration problems. Some ten years ago Dr. Tina Telakivi and a group of researchers in Finland found that snorers had subtle deficits in thinking as compared to nonsnorers. Another study, in Denmark by Drs. Poul Jennum and Anette Sjol, studied about 1,500 people and found that of self-admitted habitual snorers, *22 per-*

cent had memory problems and *57 percent* had concentration problems, much higher rates than occurred in nonsnorers. Dr. A. Jay Block and colleagues of the University of Florida and the Veterans Administration Medical Center in Gainesville gave a series of tests to sixty snorers and found that those who had the worst snoring had the worst scores the next day on IQ tests, memory, verbal fluency, reaction times, and visual coordination, and the worst recall of stories and images.

A study in 1996 at Avesta Hospital in Sweden showed that excessive daytime sleepiness at work occurred four times more often in snorers and *forty times* more often in sufferers of sleep apnea when compared to the general population. Snoring and sleep apnea were also associated with difficulties in concentrating, learning new tasks, and performing routine functions.

But the snorer usually believes that he or she slept well, never realizing just how disturbed the night's sleep was. Sleep-deprived people frequently misjudge their sleepiness and often do not understand why their performance is failing, or they mistakenly blame other factors for reduced performance. Sometimes snorers not only may mistakenly blame other factors for reduced performance, but they may even mistakenly be sent to psychiatrists because their doctors think there must be a psychological cause for their fatigue and irritability.

Many people have lived with lack of energy for so long, or it has crept up on them so gradually, that they do not know what "normal" feels like. Or they may think that being sleepy is just a sign of getting older. But it is not normal to fall asleep at your desk at work, or at a football game, or every time you sit down to watch a movie. Nor is it normal to have unexplained behavioral changes. You need to know what is causing this drowsiness and moodiness. When you get rid of it, you may be astonished at how you feel more wide awake, energetic, and alive.

And daytime sleepiness can be more—it can be a matter of life and death. Because if you're not fully alert, insufficient sleep can make you prone to accidents at home, at work, or on the road. There are many frightening examples.

The National Highway Traffic Safety Administration estimates, for example, that more than 100,000 crashes a year in the United States are related to driving while drowsy. In fact, latest statistics show that drowsy driving kills more young people in traffic accidents than does alcohol. The administration compares drowsy driving with drunk driving, and describes drowsy driving, like drunk driving, as risky and irresponsible. Indeed, hundreds of thousands die on highways around the world each year because someone fell asleep at the wheel. Reports from both New York and Pennsylvania indicate that nearly *half* of all fatal accidents on their roads are caused by drowsy drivers. And many drowsy drivers have near misses when they go through stop signs or sway out of their lane because of drowsiness or because they experience "gap driving," when they drive along in a trancelike state and have no memory of landmarks along the way. Undoubtedly, many of these sleepy drivers are suffering from sleep apnea.

A 1998 poll by the National Sleep Foundation found that 23 percent of those interviewed had fallen asleep at the wheel within the year! Lives are risked wherever there are tired drivers. Dr. Larry Findley and colleagues at the University of Virginia at Charlottesville used a driving simulation program in a lab to conclusively demonstrate the effect that sleep apnea has on daytime awareness. Those with sleep apnea hit more obstacles than those without apnea. Another study showed that patients with sleep apnea were more than ten times at risk for an automobile accident than licensed drivers in general.

Snoring and apnea unquestionably contribute to truck and car accidents due to excessive daytime sleepiness—and the estimated 1,500 fatalities that occur from them each year.

High Blood Pressure, Heart Disease, and Stroke

Aside from causing daytime sleepiness, memory and concentration problems, and decreased alertness, snoring has been shown by some studies to be related to many health conditions. Snoring may be related to high blood pressure, heart disease, and strokes; many sleep researchers are currently studying if and how snoring can cause these problems. There is much controversy around the issue, and a great deal of research going on to get to the truth.

In 1980 in Italy, Dr. Elio Lugaresi and coworkers found a strong link between snoring and high blood pressure and reported it in the journal *Sleep*. Several subsequent investigations carried out in the mid-1980s confirmed the relationship, thus establishing snoring as an important health hazard. However, because high blood pressure and snoring are both affected by the same factors—obesity, age, cigarette smoking—there was some doubt whether the snoring alone had an independent influence on blood pressure, or whether it affected it indirectly because it was associated with these other factors. In addition, many of the people with high blood pressure who snored turned out to also have sleep apnea along with their snoring, and so it could have been the apnea that was linked to the high blood pressure.

A study conducted by Dr. Terry Young and others at the University of Wisconsin at Madison analyzed data from 580 people and found that people with snoring, even without apnea, were significantly at risk of high blood pressure, with the risk becoming greater as the snoring became worse, and most severe when apneas appeared. And in other studies, even when weight and smoking and other factors were taken into account, researchers found that people who are habitual snorers are more likely to have high blood pressure, and in fact, when these people were treated for their snoring, their blood pressure returned to normal.

There was, and still is, controversy also about the relationship of snoring to heart disease and strokes. Some studies indicate that snoring is associated with these outcomes, while other studies do not confirm this association. It is still too premature to give a simple yes or no to the question of whether there is a relationship between snoring and vascular disease. But some researchers believe that many people who die in their sleep may have had a heart attack or stroke brought on by the complications of heavy snoring and the stopped-breathing episodes of apnea often associated with such snoring.

Other Health Problems

In addition to all these problems, several studies have shown that heavy snorers have other problems, for example, frequent bad morning headaches.

If there is apnea, oxygen levels in the blood are lowered, causing additional problems. For example, the *Journal of Sex and Marital Therapy* reports that sexual dysfunction in men can be related to chronic decreased oxygen at night.

Also some early small studies suggest the possibility that loud snoring, like other loud noises, might lead to hearing loss, and indeed might be the cause of some of the "normal" hearing loss that sometimes occurs with age. The first report about this was in 1973 by Dr. M.

Prazic of the University of Zagreb in Yugoslavia. He compared the pillow-level noise of snoring to the noise heard by a worker in a noisy factory. "A snorer snores usually every night for several hours for years, even decades," he wrote. "It would be difficult to presume that no damage of the snorer's hearing took place." He examined seventeen snorers and found that they all had measurable hearing losses. It may not be a coincidence that the wife of the man awarded the title of snoring champion (i.e., the loudest snorer) in 1992 became deaf in one ear.

Snoring Can Be Treated

Snoring is not just a social nuisance; it is an important medical condition. It can be connected to other medical problems and it can cause medical problems on its own.

But despite snoring's prevalence, and despite its effect on daytime quality of life and its medical importance, very few people get treated. In fact, they seldom even think of the possibility of treatment, and physicians seldom ask about sleep patterns or snoring, or suggest treatment.

We consider the impact of snoring and apnea on health and well-being to be so significant that we believe that as part of every checkup physicians should ask patients if they snore or have been told they stop breathing when sleeping or have other sleep problems. If their physician doesn't bring up the subject, then any person who has the problems should bring the subject up.

You don't have to tolerate the sleep-robbing racket in your bedroom, or the health complications from snoring. There are many treatments for snoring now available. Researchers have learned much in the last few years, such as the fact that most snoring can be cured by the lifestyle changes of losing weight, avoiding alcohol, sleeping pills, and muscle relaxants, and quitting smoking, and that more severe cases can be cured with dental appliances, breathing aids, and new techniques of simple surgery. Unfortunately, the news has mostly not been reaching the public.

We hope this book will change that. We'll discuss the many different causes of snoring and the dangerous things that can make your snoring worse, and help you learn more about your particular problem with snoring, the possible causes in your case, and the specific things that you can do for your best treatment.

It brings together advice from doctors at St. Michael's Hospital and the University of Toronto, and from other researchers and specialists around the world to give you an integrated, step-by-step no-more-snoring program to treat *your* snoring problems. We give you advice on simple lifestyle changes and other remedies that can help your snoring as well as information on the latest techniques, appliances, and surgery. We tell you about different remedies, help you answer questions about your snoring, and tell you what step-by-step things you can do to help you with your particular problem. Follow the steps in the program, and you may be able to put an end to the noisy nights that keep others awake, the tired days after sleep-disturbed nights, and the hidden health problems that may be gradually affecting your body.

The programs at St. Michael's Hospital and other sleep disorders centers work. The success rate at St. Michael's for patients who comply with the program is over 90 percent. And there is a long waiting list.

But first, just as would happen if you came to the sleep disorders center at St. Michael's Hospital and the University of Toronto, we want to answer some of the most common questions and in so doing tell you some facts and controversies about snoring. We'll do that in the next chapter.

2

The Facts about Snoring and Sleep Apnea

Before we get into the best treatments for snoring, here are some answers to common questions that will give you the facts to help you understand your problem better.

What Is Snoring?

There are different kinds of snoring and different causes for snoring. For example, snoring is especially likely to occur in people who have broken noses, who are overweight, or who have short fat necks. It may be a symptom of a cold or the stuffed-up nasal passages of hayfever. It may be a result of loose muscles in the throat from the relaxation caused by alcohol, sleeping pills, or tranquilizers. It may be due to being fat, which causes loose tissue in the throat to flap around just like the loose tissue on the rest of the body. Or it can be a symptom of a thyroid problem, a tumor, or a neuromuscular disease affecting the tone of upper airway muscles. Some patients start snoring after having a stroke that affects their speech and swallowing or that causes vocal cord paralysis.

Some people snore every night, all night; others snore only when they first fall asleep or when they are in deep sleep, or when they sleep on their back, or under special circumstances like when they have a cold or have had too much to drink.

It used to be thought that a snore happens only when a person breathes in. Now researchers have learned that a snore can occur in both inhalation and exhalation. It mostly happens when the person's mouth is open, but it can occur also when breathing through the nose or through the nose and mouth combined. Some people snore breathing in, then when breathing out produce a puffing sound from the lips. (Scientists who love big words have named this phenomenon *explosive labial exhalation.*)

Snoring can occur anytime during sleep, but studies in sleep laboratories show that it occurs most often in the deeper stages of sleep, and sometimes during dreaming. Usually people who snore don't get enough deep sleep, one of the reasons for fatigue the next day.

What Actually Happens When You Snore?

The tissues of the throat are soft and collapsible, and during sleep their muscle tone is diminished even more. What usually happens during snoring is that a vibration is produced in the tissues of the throat. Sometimes the vibration is in the region of the uvula, that little bit of tissue that you can see hanging down in the back of your throat. Or there can be vibrations lower down, involving tissue in the back of the throat, at the base of the tongue or near the opening of the throat to the bronchial tubes.

The airway from your nose and mouth to your throat and down to your lungs is like a wind tunnel. When you inhale forcefully, the entire throat–trachea–bronchial-tube wind tunnel is lengthened and pulled downward, resulting in a narrowing of the airway. Imagine some loose panels in there—when a rush of air comes through, those panels are going to rattle. If you have an obstruction in the airway, or if the airway is narrowed because you have a small throat or mouth, or because of excess tissue or irritation or swelling, or because your tongue falls back toward your throat—whatever the reason—it narrows the wind tunnel, increases the force of the air coming through, and makes the vibrations stronger.

There is also an effect called *Bernoulli's principle* (remember high school physics?): When there is increased airflow through a hollow tube, it produces a drop in pressure. This pulls the throat tissue inward, making it narrower and adding to the vibration.

The bottom line: a snoring sound is produced from the combination of a narrowed cross-sectional area of the wind tunnel, the floppiness of its walls, and the flow of air through it. The narrower the airway, the stronger the rush of air, and the stronger the vibration and the snore.

It is important to understand this fundamental principle, because it will help you to understand the various strategies we will tell you later for treatment of snoring. All of the treatments will be directed either to increasing the cross-sectional area of the airway, increasing the stiffness of the airway walls, or reducing the force of the flow of air through the airway.

Snoring can be produced in different locations along the airway in different people. In fact, the vibration can occur at any point inside the wind tunnel, anywhere along the airway. In fact, even in the same person, snoring may be generated at different sites at different times.

The first opportunity for production of snoring is by obstruction in the nose. When you breathe through your nose, the air must go through two narrow openings only about one-tenth of an inch wide in the back of each nostril.

Many nose conditions can narrow the airway. You may have a deviated septum if your nose has been broken. You may have had surgery that resulted in thickening and scarring of tissues that reduced the area of the nasal passage. Or you may have nasal polyps plugging up your nose. Swelling of the nasal tissues can also result from an allergy, pregnancy, a cold, or overuse of nasal sprays. (Overuse of decongestant nasal sprays can cause congestion as a rebound reaction.) And many irritants in the air, especially cigarette smoke, can increase airway congestion and cause or increase the severity of snoring.

Whatever the reason, if your nasal passages are narrow, you have to breathe harder and use more effort to get the amount of air you need to provide your body with oxygen and to wash out carbon dioxide. This increased effort alone can lead to vibrations of the wind tunnel wall and produce snoring.

In addition, usually with each inhalation of breath, a partial vacuum is formed drawing in air. That vacuum exerts a pulling effect on the tissues, and if the tissues in the throat are limp and the air comes through with more force, then the throat tissue can vibrate more or even close.

This is not all just theory, by the way. The various snoring sites have actually been seen vibrating by investigators looking into the airway through a fiberoptic videoscope during sleep.

Snoringlike noise production also was shown rather neatly in a model constructed with an elastic tube by two researchers, Drs. Noam Gavriely of the Rappaport Institute for Research in Medicine in Israel and Oliver Jensen of the University of Newcastle upon Tyne in Great Britain. They found that airflow through the tube could make the tube walls begin to vibrate and generate noises that sounded remarkably like those produced when humans snore.

Wherever your snore is generated, the tone and the loudness of the snore will depend on how much air is going through, how fast and forcefully the air is traveling, how much flabby tissue there is, and how much the tissue vibrates.

The potential for narrowing of the airway is greatest during sleep because your tongue and throat muscles become more relaxed then. This is why drinking alcohol can make snoring so much worse—it relaxes muscle tissue and causes the tongue to drop even more into the back of the throat. Sleeping pills and tranquilizers also cause muscle relaxation, and may also decrease nerve impulses going to the upper airway muscles, thus making the walls of the airway even more limp. Badly fitting dentures are often a hidden factor, too—they strain the mouth muscles in the daytime, and when the dentures are removed at night, the muscles relax more than they would ordinarily.

And there are other things that can narrow the airway. You may have fat deposits in your throat that narrow the passageway. You may have an enlarged tongue or an enlarged uvula, or you may have enlarged tonsils and adenoids, the frequent cause of snoring in children. You may have an incorrectly positioned jaw or a receding chin. Neck size is also significant—snorers on average have bigger necks than nonsnorers.

Because there are so many causes of snoring and so many things that can make it worse, you need an integrated program that includes all facets of the various causes and the treatments for them.

How Loud Can Snoring Get?

Very. A little night music isn't always so little. Some patients who were referred to the University of Toronto sleep laboratory because of snoring registered a sound in excess of 100 decibels, about the same as a motorcycle running. (A pneumatic drill registers about 110 decibels.)

A decibel is the measurement of the intensity of a sound, with zero

decibels as the quietest sound heard by a normal human ear. Ten decibels would be like the rustle of leaves in a light breeze; 20 decibels, like
an average whisper. One hundred decibels is closer to the sound of
a passing jet. Some doctors use a less scientific rating system of snoring—based on the number of doors that have to be closed to escape
the noise.

President Theodore Roosevelt was known to be a very loud snorer,
and the story is told that he once snored so loudly in a hospital that
complaints were filed by almost every patient in the wing where he was
recuperating. Winston Churchill, too, was a loud snorer. In Cincinnati
a man was sent to jail for stealing, but soon after being jailed, his snoring was so bad that the other prisoners couldn't sleep at night, and the
warden said the snoring prisoner couldn't stay awake on any job given
him. They released him.

One patient—Paul—who came to St. Michael's was a loud snorer.
He loved fishing and camping, and when he would go every autumn
with his buddies, they would set up a large tent where everyone would
sleep in their sleeping bags. Except Paul. He snored so loudly that they
wouldn't let him sleep in the same tent and made him set up his own
tent away from theirs. His sleep test later in the lab showed that he
did not have sleep apnea, but that he snored loudly and frequently
throughout the night. His maximum snoring sound registered at 100
decibels, and even the average sound during the night registered at 85
decibels.

One 66-year-old man came to the clinic, one of the loudest snorers
the clinic had ever come across. How loud was he? For years his wife
slept in a different room because of the noise. When they moved into a
new neighborhood, they regularly got complaints about his snoring
from the next-door neighbors! In fact, his snoring was audible in the
house across the street whenever bedroom windows were open. His
snoring sound registered at 110 decibels.

Who Snores Most? and When?

If you snore, you're not alone. Snoring occurs at all ages and all over
the world, in both men and women, and even in children.

Sleep experts know that snoring is very common, but can only provide estimates of the actual numbers and percentages of people who

snore. The usual number quoted for the United States is that some 88 million adults snore to some degree, and more than a third of them snore regularly, usually every night.

The percentages of snorers reported by different surveys made in different countries show huge variations—from 10 to 86 percent of men, and from 7 to 57 percent of women.

Why the differences in different surveys? There sometimes were differences in how the questions were phrased, in methods used, and in the segments or ages of the people who were interviewed. Some questionnaires dealt with any snoring, others with only severe snoring.

Also, snoring is heard differently by different listeners—different people listening at the same time to the same person snoring will perceive the sound differently. Snorers themselves usually don't hear their own snoring. Some say that they occasionally are awakened during the night by their own snoring, but most are unaware of their snoring and deny vehemently that they snore at all. One investigator, Dr. John Stradling of Oxford, England, asked almost 1,000 men whether they snored, and found that the prevalence of snoring more than doubled when wives were present during the interview and contributed to the information.

Men versus Women

In most surveys, snoring is about twice as common in men as in women, particularly premenopausal women. We're not sure why. One possibility is that female hormones may help protect the throat muscles from becoming floppy and vibrating during sleep, one of the causes of snoring. Studies have shown that giving the female hormone progesterone to men can reduce their snoring and also sleep apnea, whereas testosterone can increase airway resistance in women. Another possibility is that men may not be as aware of their bedpartners' snoring and do not report it as frequently. Pregnant women snore more than nonpregnant women, perhaps because they have more swelling of tissue in the upper airway during the third trimester, or perhaps due to weight gain.

Age and Snoring

There are very few studies examining what happens to snorers as they grow older. The likelihood of snoring seems to increase with age. In a study in Cleveland, habitual snoring was reported by 14 percent of adults younger than 25 years, and increased to 46 percent in adults over age 50. In a study done by Dr. Terry Young and other researchers at the University of Wisconsin, habitual snoring was reported by 35 percent of men aged 30–39, and increased to 53 percent for men in the 50–60 age group. However, after age 65, snoring seems to occur less frequently.

Studies in Finland and at the University of Arizona and St. Michael's show that in many people, snoring becomes worse over the years. But that can be stopped or even reversed by eliminating lifestyle habits that encourage snoring. For example, if you snore habitually, but manage to lose weight and have no respiratory symptoms, such as cough, phlegm, or wheezing, there is at least a 30 percent chance that your snoring will go away. On the other hand, if you only snore occasionally and make no changes in your unhealthy habits, there is a 10 to 15 percent chance that your snoring will worsen and you will become a habitual snorer.

By the way, snoring can occur in children, too. Seven percent of newborn babies have injuries to the nose from delivery, which can cause snoring. Children often snore if they have a stuffy nose from an allergy or cold. Or they may snore because they have enlarged tonsils and adenoids, or even a bean, a piece of candy, or some other foreign object stuffed up the nose.

Sleep apnea can have a profound influence on a child's life. One review showed that of 100 children with confirmed sleep apnea, 73 had excessive daytime sleepiness noted by parents and teachers, more than half had nightmares or night terrors, many had morning headaches, and most were markedly underweight for their age and had poor school performance. Nighttime problems included bedwetting, sleepwalking, excessive sweating, restlessness, and frequent awakenings.

Why Is Snoring Worse When You Lie on Your Back?

When you lie on your back, your jaw usually opens, your tongue and soft palate (the soft part at the back of the roof of your mouth) shift closer to the back wall of the throat, thus narrowing the airway. You must exert more effort to draw air through the narrowed airway, so the air comes through with more force. Because of the force and the suction created, the airway and the throat tissues collapse and vibrate even more than usual.

In addition, if you're lying on your back, fluid can accumulate in the blood vessels around the narrow nasal passages, which makes breathing through the nose more difficult.

If you are a heavy snorer, you may also snore when on your side. This happens because there is still some narrowing of the cross-sectional area of the throat whenever you lie down in any position. In addition, you may have to breathe harder because your nose is partly congested. When you sleep, there is a normal cycle of alternating congestion and decongestion of the nostrils that occurs in about 75 percent of people, and which can affect nasal resistance and cause snoring. The duration of the cycle varies a lot; it can be as short as fifteen minutes in some people, or as long as several hours in others. Not much is known yet about this rather weird phenomenon, but usually it is the nostril on your "down" side which becomes congested first. When this happens, you usually turn over onto the opposite side for relief so that the breathing is unobstructed for a while, but then the "down" nostril becomes congested again, and the cycle repeats itself.

Is Snoring Hereditary?

Many snorers report that one or both of their parents snored loudly. Indeed, there are now several studies suggesting that snoring may sometimes involve a hereditary factor. For example, Dr. Poul Jennum and his colleagues in Denmark administered questionnaires to more than 3,000 men in Copenhagen asking about their own snoring as well as snoring among their grandparents, parents, brothers, sisters, and children. They found a strong relationship between snoring and a family history of snoring. Habitual snorers were about three times more likely than nonsnorers to have family members who also snored habitually.

In another study, Dr. Luigi Ferrini-Strambi and colleagues at the sleep disorders center of the State University of Milan asked 386 pairs of twins in Italy (some identical and some nonidentical) about their snoring habits. They found that if one of the identical twins snored, there was a 67 percent chance that the other identical twin also snored. Among nonidentical twins, the chance was only 50 percent.

In France, Dr. Dan Teculescu and his colleagues questioned parents of children who snored and found a strong association between the children's snoring and snoring by a family member. Similar studies were done by Dr. Susan Redline of Rhode Island and colleagues at several centers throughout the United States, as well as by Dr. Christian Guilleminault and colleagues at Stanford University. Both groups found that patients who snored and had apnea were more likely than non-snorers to have family members who snored. But most of them were also overweight.

Based on the information we have to date, it appears that snoring and apnea have a strong hereditary component. However, interaction with environmental factors (obesity, smoking, alcohol, a broken nose) will have a major influence on the hereditary predisposition to snoring. Whether you lose weight or control another major risk factor in snoring is just as important as whether you come from a family of snorers.

What about Other Sleeptime Noises?

All breathing noises are not snoring. Two very common chronic diseases—asthma and chronic bronchitis—may cause breathing noises during sleep. A high-pitched musical sound is characteristic of asthma. A low-pitched sound with cough, phlegm, and shortness of breath is characteristic of bronchitis (usually caused by cigarette smoking). A barking sound may be a sign of respiratory infection, such as whooping cough or pneumonia. Children with croup will very frequently make a sound, called *stridor*, that may sound like snoring. Some adults with neuromuscular diseases causing dysfunction or paralysis of the vocal cords will also produce an extremely loud sound when breathing in.

A 47-year-old woman came to the clinic whose husband complained that she recently had started snoring very loudly, disturbing the sleep of all the other members of the family. During her initial interview she said she had also noticed changes in her voice, and she had become hoarse. In addition, her energy level had decreased and she had begun to feel tired during the day. Snoring and daytime tiredness are characteristic of sleep apnea, and that is why she was referred to our clinic. But this woman had not gained weight; there was no obvious change in her lifestyle or medications to explain the rapid onset of her snoring and her hoarseness. She was referred to a neurologist, who found that she had a neurological disorder that involved her larynx muscles so that her vocal cords were partially paralyzed, narrowing during sleep and producing the noise that her family perceived as snoring. Eventually the woman developed complete paralysis of her vocal cords and obstruction of her upper airway, and surgery had to be performed to correct her problem.

You need to remember also that a person can have more than one condition, and might snore as well as make the noises of asthma, bronchitis, emphysema, or other conditions. Or you may hear people grind their teeth, which can cause not only daytime sleepiness from so many awakenings but also an aching jaw or headache in the morning.

Do Those Who Lie and Listen Also Suffer?

Definitely. Snoring affects the person sleeping in the same room or the same bed—sometimes the same house! In one survey almost two-thirds of the people surveyed who were living with a snorer said they lost sleep each week because of the noise. More than half said they probably lost up to two hours of sleep a night, and some said they lost more sleep than that.

And they weren't happy. Most of them were annoyed, angry, and resentful that they had to listen to the noise and lose sleep.

The impact of snoring and apnea upon a marriage can be horrendous. Several studies have been done looking at the effect of snoring on the person living with the snorer and on marriages. Drs. Rosalind Cartwright and Sara Knight, of Rush-Presbyterian–St. Luke's Medical Center in Chicago, studied male patients with sleep apnea who had been referred to their sleep laboratory because of snoring. The patients and the wives were interviewed and also asked to fill out several standard questionnaires for assessing mood. Many slept in separate bedrooms or separate beds. The wives said they were irritated and worried about their husband's snoring, and because of the husband's daytime sleepiness, they were lonely, disappointed, angry, and frustrated. The husband-patients were depressed, exhausted, and felt socially isolated.

One 34-year-old man went to a doctor because of his snoring. Married five years, his wife complained bitterly about his snoring, which had become worse during the previous year when he had a 35-pound weight gain. At first she tried earplugs, but she was still awakened by his loud snoring. Then she tried sleeping in the next room with the door closed, but found that even this did not protect her from the noise. Then she had the basement renovated, two flights below the master bedroom, so she could have somewhere to escape when he snored. He was eventually referred to St. Michael's Hospital and was found to have sleep apnea. He was treated, lost weight, and got rid of both his snoring and his apnea. However, he and his wife did not live happily ever after and got divorced for other reasons after two years.

Not only can snoring separate spouses during sleeptime, but because of the snorer's fatigue it can also cut into their shared time during the day and evening. This occurs so often that Dr. Cartwright suggests that because of the extended stress on the marital and family unit, a support group be started for partners and family members of patients who severely snore or have sleep apnea.

Drs. William Beninati and John Shepard Jr. of the sleep disorders center at Mayo Clinic in Rochester, Minnesota, termed this disturbance and sleep fragmentation of the snorer's bedpartner the "spousal arousal syndrome." They reported at the 1997 meeting of the American Sleep Disorders Association on ten people who had sleep apnea and their spouses. The person with apnea was studied for half the night with CPAP treatment to eliminate the apnea and half the night without the treatment. (We will explain this treatment in a later chapter.) They counted the number of arousals from sleep and sleep efficiency of the person *without* apnea and found that when the apnea patient was treated with CPAP, the partner without apnea had fewer arousals, and thus less fragmented sleep.

So things can get better. In 1997 Drs. James Kiely and Walter McNicholas of Dublin, Ireland, questioned the bedpartners of patients who had apnea and snored. When the apnea and snoring were treated and abolished, the bedpartners said they were less sleepy and tired during the day and they had better interpersonal relationships with their partners.

What Does It Mean If a Person Sometimes Stops Breathing?

Your spouse lies there snoring, snoring, snoring—then suddenly the snoring stops, *his breathing stops!*—you wait and wait and wait, and finally it starts up again with a gasp and a snort. This is apnea.

The term *apnea* is Greek and means the absence of breathing. An episode of apnea is considered to occur when you don't breathe for ten seconds or more. It can sometimes even last longer, more than a minute. The sleeper might not be aware of it, but the bedpartner probably is because it can be really scary to hear someone suddenly stop breathing and then start snorting and gasping for air, and sometimes thrash about.

An episode of a partial reduction of airflow to less than 50 percent of the person's normal breathing is called *hypopnea* (as opposed to the total absence of airflow in apnea).

A person with typical apnea or hypopnea will have episodes of completely or partially stopped breathing that last ten seconds or longer, and will have ten or more such episodes per hour. Some people may have up to several hundred apnea and hypopnea episodes each night. An occasional episode of apnea is quite common, and fewer than a total of ten episodes of apnea and hypopnea per hour is considered normal. In some people, even this mild apnea activity can interrupt sleep enough to cause tiredness and sleepiness the next day. If you have any abnormal breathing and feel tired and sleepy, talk to your doctor about it.

The severity of a person's stopped-breathing episodes is measured by what doctors call the *apnea-hypopnea index (AHI)*, which is the average number of total episodes of both apnea and hypopnea during one hour of sleep. It is also called the *respiratory disturbance index (RDI)*. The higher the RDI (or AHI) number, the more severe the apnea.

Then, to make it confusing, you need to know that there are actually two types of apnea. In one type, *central apnea*, the airway stays partially open, but the respiratory center in your brain fails to send the appropriate signal to the breathing muscles of the diaphragm and chest; in other words, the drive to breathe is not activated. You eventually awaken for lack of air. Central apnea is relatively rare; it sometimes follows strokes, or may be part of postpolio syndrome or a symptom of heart failure, or may occur after a brain injury.

The most common form of apnea is *obstructive sleep apnea (OSA)*. It is called "obstructive" because the stoppage of breathing is due to a repetitive collapse and obstruction of the airway. This form of apnea occurs when the upper airway is blocked. The blockage may be due to a uvula that is very large or a tongue that is set too far back in the mouth so that it is sucked in when you inhale. Or it may be that the airway is so small and flaccid that it doesn't just vibrate as it would when simply snoring, but gets completely sucked closed. There is also some evidence that the airways of people with apnea are more likely to collapse because they are unusually shaped and are more collapsible than the airways of people who don't have apnea.

During obstructive sleep apnea, the airway is blocked and no air flows, but the person still attempts to breathe. The diaphragm and chest muscles work to expand the lungs and draw in the air, but the throat is so completely blocked that no air passes through. Because the body is getting no air, the oxygen level in the person's blood drops, and the carbon dioxide level rises; then after a few seconds, because of the low oxygen and high carbon dioxide level in the blood, an arousal signal is sent from the brain, which momentarily awakens the person. During this arousal, the muscles of the tongue and throat tighten, which helps to reopen the airway, and with a loud snort or gasp, the person takes a breath again. Usually the awakening is so brief it isn't remembered, but the repeated awakenings all through the night can keep the person from getting a good night's sleep.

There is also *mixed apnea,* where you have a little of both kinds of apnea.

To confuse everyone even more, the terminology police decided that there is a difference between the terms *obstructive sleep apnea (OSA)* and *obstructive sleep apnea syndrome (OSAS),* sometimes also called *sleep apnea syndrome (SAS).* OSA in its strictest sense means laboratory demonstration of a certain number of episodes of apnea and hypopnea per hour of sleep, without necessarily any daytime symptoms such as sleepiness or fatigue. OSAS or SAS, on the other hand, means laboratory demonstration of episodes of apnea and hypopnea with daytime symptoms.

Another term, *sleep-disordered breathing (SDB),* can refer to any breathing abnormalities during sleep; for example, there is a crescendo-decrescendo pattern of breathing called *Cheyne-Stokes respiration,* sometimes seen in patients with heart failure or stroke. But since sleep apnea is the most common breathing abnormality during sleep, SDB is most often used to denote sleep apnea.

It all sounds confusing, but all you need to remember is that stopped breathing is apnea and partially reduced breathing is hypopnea. And either one can cause you to be tired the next day as well as cause many other medical problems.

Can Apnea Be Life-Threatening?

Yes, and in several ways. Apnea can be responsible for an astounding number of problems.

Because of the constant disruption of sleep and the low oxygen levels, people with apnea often have early-morning headaches, then fatigue during the day. And sometimes they also suffer from memory losses, irritability, depression, learning difficulty, impotence, and other sexual dysfunction. Indeed, sleep apnea can impair brain function, not just because it causes daytime sleepiness, but because it actually damages the brain. Think of the countless episodes when the brain's oxygen supply is reduced, time after time, night after night. It's bound to eventually take its toll.

Some research indicates that there is a possibility that apnea also might be implicated in sudden infant death syndrome, and more research is being carried out in this area.

One of the biggest problems caused by nighttime apnea is the resulting uncontrollable daytime sleepiness. Some patients describe it as being like permanent jet lag. The sleepiness is often a cause of lack of concentration on the job and reduced energy levels that can negatively affect one's career and social life.

And apnea-caused sleepiness has now been cited as a hidden cause of automobile accidents. The most recent studies show not only that people in whom sleep apnea has been diagnosed have more car accidents than those without, but that those with most severe apnea have the highest rate of accidents. In many states and provinces, physicians have a legal obligation to report to the licensing authorities their driving patients suspected of having sleep apnea. Auto accidents are so common in patients with sleep apnea that many sleep clinics advise their patients not to drive until they have received treatment.

Also as we pointed out earlier, sleep apnea appears to be a factor in high blood pressure, heart disease, and stroke. In fact, it has been estimated that up to 30 percent of sleep apnea patients have high blood pressure. Normally, blood pressure decreases during sleep. But according to the results of many researchers, sleep apnea patients often experience an *increase* in blood pressure during sleep following each apnea episode. Furthermore, to quote from a position statement issued by the American Sleep Apnea Association, "this increase occurs just as blood oxygen levels may be falling, creating a potential crisis for sleep apnea patients with heart disease." High blood pressure is found in more than half of all apnea patients, and patients with apnea also have a high frequency of heart arrhythmia. By some estimates, as many as 90 percent of apnea patients have slowed heartbeats, long pauses, extra beats, and other types of mix-ups in rhythm.

It is difficult for the heart to beat when oxygen saturation in the blood is low and air pressure in the lungs is fluctuating wildly. When oxygen levels fall, the heart works harder to get oxygen to the brain. The lower the level of saturation, the greater the chance that heart problems will occur. Normally, the oxygen saturation level is 90 percent or greater during sleep. If levels drop to 85 percent or lower, there is usually an increase in pulmonary artery blood pressure, which can put a strain on the heart and eventually lead to heart failure. Heart arrhythmia or stopping of the heart can occur, especially if the oxygen saturation level of the blood falls below 60 percent.

In a study by Drs. Markku Partinen and Christian Guilleminault of Stanford University, sleep apnea patients had twice the prevalence of high blood pressure, three times as much heart disease, and four times as much brain circulatory disease as others. Another study, in Australia, found that patients hospitalized for heart attack were many times more likely to have sleep apnea than others. The authors of the study suggest that sleep apnea increases the risk of heart attack by up to twenty-five times.

In fact, an estimated 38,000 cardiovascular deaths annually are directly attributable to sleep apnea, according to the National Commission on Sleep Disorders Research. And apnea may be responsible for $3 million to $2 billion of the health care costs associated with the treatment of heart disease and stroke.

Apnea, like the simple snoring that often precedes it, can occur at any age, but is more common in older people. Most people over age 75 have an occasional stopped-breathing episode. In one study the prevalence of significant sleep apnea among nursing home residents was found to be 42 percent, with half of these having apnea so severe as to be life-threatening. In that and other studies, Dr. Sonia Ancoli-Israel and her colleagues of San Diego found that apnea not only increased the risk of death of patients in nursing homes but sometimes was responsible for making their dementia symptoms worse.

"He just died in his sleep" may sound like a merciful way to go, but dying in your sleep could often be an unnecessary death caused by the complications of hidden or untreated apnea.

Why Is Apnea Often Not Diagnosed?

Unfortunately, few physicians talk to their patients about snoring or apnea, and as a result most patients with the problem are still not being treated. In fact, even as recently as 1997 an article in *Archives of Internal Medicine,* a journal of the American Medical Association, reported that sleep apnea is a significant public health problem and that it is "dramatically unrecognized by primary care physicians." Dr. Eric Ball of the Walla Walla Clinic in Walla Walla, Washington, said in the article that his and his colleagues' research indicated that the majority of Americans' sleep disorders remain undiagnosed and untreated.

The typical sleep apnea patient experiences symptoms for five to ten years before seeking medical attention! In a 1997 report, Dr. John Ronald and other researchers at St. Boniface General Hospital Research Center and the University of Manitoba in Canada said that in their study of patient records they found that sleep apnea patients used health care resources at about twice the rate of others as much as ten years before diagnosis, and had more physician care and more hospitalizations.

Yet when apnea sufferers go to their doctors, the condition is many times not diagnosed, and often mistakenly called insomnia and treated with sleeping pills that make apnea worse. In 1993 one computer search of medical records showed that of more than 10 million patients seen by physicians in the United States in 1989 and 1990, sleep apnea was diagnosed in only 73 patients.

People with apnea sometimes view their problem as insomnia since their sleep is so restless, and they may take sleeping pills, which only makes the problem worse by further depressing the central nervous system. This is potentially very dangerous. If you have been found to have more than ten apnea episodes per hour, we urge you not to take sleeping pills unless your doctor says you have some special condition that requires it.

The truth is that people with serious apnea are at risk of dying of its complications if it is not treated!

Fortunately, the picture is now changing, with new medical focus being placed on apnea and other sleep disorders and extensive medical education being conducted on the subject, and with the growth in the number of sleep disorders centers, which has risen from 164 in 1990 to more than 300 today.

Interestingly, it is often when a person is widowed or divorced, then remarries, that apnea is discovered—by the second spouse. The threat of separate beds often gets the victim to the doctor, and what may have been interpreted as nagging turns out to be lifesaving.

And sometimes apnea is diagnosed, but the patient doesn't take the symptoms and the doctor's advice seriously. In the book *No More Sleepless Nights* (by Drs. Peter Hauri and Shirley Linde), a case was described of a 45-year-old man who was severely obese (313 pounds) and who complained of always being sleepy during the day. He had previously been a successful businessman, but later was never able to hold a job for more than two or three weeks because of his falling asleep on the job five to ten times a day. He had seen many doctors, and spent more than $200,000 trying to find a cause for his sleepiness. Two wives left him. He couldn't maintain social relationships with friends because he was always sleepy. Tests in the sleep lab showed heavy snoring and more than 500 episodes of apnea through the night. More than 75 percent of his "sleep" was spent not breathing! He declined recommended treatment for "a mere sleep problem." He became a heavy drinker and a year later died in his sleep of "unknown causes."

If you have loud snoring or many stopped-breathing episodes, or both, and you also have excessive daytime sleepiness, go to a doctor and discuss your symptoms. If he does not investigate your symptoms or prescribes sleeping pills, go to another doctor. Sleep apnea can have deadly results if untreated.

Who Gets Apnea?

Prevalence rates for sleep apnea differ for men and women and are estimated to be about 10 percent for men and 5 percent for women. The number of people who have it is in the millions. Men are more commonly affected by apnea than women, perhaps due to the protective effect of progesterone in premenopausal women; however, in postmenopausal women this protective effect is no longer present, and the prevalence of sleep apnea among women begins to approach that of men.

Apnea can occur in children, too. Such children often are thought to be lazy or dumb, when they are really very tired from never sleeping well. So if your young child or teenager seems sleepy or lazy, listen at night for heavy snoring or pauses in breathing. Sometimes the awakenings at night from apnea also cause a problem with bedwetting. Several studies have shown that if enlarged tonsils are causing the apnea, then removing the tonsils will sometimes cure the bedwetting.

Apnea, like snoring, can run in families.

Unfortunately, the patient often does not know there is a problem. Many older people, for example, live alone and no one observes the apnea. Others may not believe it when told. If you snore a lot, you should consider the possibility of sleep apnea. (We will tell you how to check for it and do other at-home tests in the next chapter.) It is important to see a doctor for consultation and an evaluation of your condition, and to get help especially if you have daytime sleepiness or a heart condition.

What Is the Relationship between Snoring and Apnea?

Snoring and apnea may be part of a continuous spectrum. First, the person has mild snoring, then increasingly more severe snoring, then perhaps snoring with difficulty in getting enough air. Then the person may experience some of the stopped-breathing episodes of apnea, followed by serious apnea with excessive daytime sleepiness. Finally, cardiovascular complications may occur. That's the way many researchers see it—a continuous spectrum of problems in varying degrees from mild to severe, with snoring progressively leading to apnea. Dr. Elio Lugaresi of Bologna, Italy, was the first researcher to suggest this, and coined the term "heavy snorer's disease," with four stages of disease leading from snoring to apnea.

Some people are between stages. They may struggle to get air during the night and snore, and may be sleepy and tired during the day, but they do not have episodes of apnea or hypopnea. These people are nonapneic snorers, and the term *upper airway resistance syndrome* has been given to their problem.

Dr. Eliot Phillipson at the University of Toronto wrote of the possible gradual pattern from snoring to apnea in an editorial in the *New England Journal of Medicine*. "Complete airway collapse during sleep is usually preceded by years of narrowing that produces snoring," he wrote. "Thus, by the time adults with obstructive sleep apnea come to medical attention, they have a long history of loud snoring, often beginning in childhood."

"Ten to 15 years ago obstructive sleep apnea was considered to be a medical curiosity that was of little importance," Dr. Phillipson wrote in the journal. "As noted by the National Commission on Sleep Disorders Research, it is time for the nation to wake up to the staggering impact of sleep disturbances on the health and welfare of our society; an impact that rivals that of smoking."

According to the National Commission on Sleep Disorders Research, obstructive sleep apnea, untreated, will have a progressive, unremitting course and can lead to fatal complications. However, we do not know yet how often untreated snoring leads to sleep apnea. No long-term studies have followed nonapneic snorers to see how many develop apnea. We do know that untreated snoring leading to apnea is plausible, since apnea becomes more common as you grow older. One would therefore expect that nonapneic snorers will eventually develop apnea as they get older. And we do know that a snorer who drinks alcohol or gains weight is at a higher risk of developing sleep apnea than a nonsnorer doing the same things.

Can Apnea Be Treated?

Yes, many things will help apnea sufferers.

The person with apnea should avoid the use of alcohol and tobacco, which make the airway more likely to collapse during sleep. Certain medicines should be avoided also, such as sleeping pills and muscle relaxants or any medicine that causes relaxation of muscles. Overweight people can benefit from losing weight, even if only ten to twenty pounds. And there are different medical and surgical treatments, with recommendations depending on how severe the apnea is and other factors. We'll tell you about all the treatments for snoring and apnea in later chapters.

3

Testing Yourself at Home

Some people snore softly, while others sound like a jackhammer next to your ear, driving away bedpartners and frightening small children. Some snort and hack, some rumble, some hiss or whistle. Some snore every night, others only occasionally. Some snore only when lying on their backs, others when they eat too much or too late, or when they drink too much. Then there are those who snore because they smoke, because their throat tissue is fat or loose, because they are having an unrealized reaction to a medication, or because they have an allergy.

There are many things that can influence snoring and its severity. Different things can affect different people, and different things can be an influence at different times, even in the same person.

There are several simple things that you can check at home to determine whether you snore, what your snoring sounds like, how severe it is, what factors might be causing your snoring, and whether you also have the stopped-breathing episodes of apnea. Finding out some of these things will not only help you understand how serious your snoring is, but will also help you learn what aspects of your own lifestyle could be contributing to your problem. That way, you will know where to concentrate your efforts to conquer your snoring.

It is important to understand the underlying cause or causes of your snoring in order to find the best and most targeted treatment. Otherwise, you may end up doing expensive and inappropriate things aimed at the wrong target. Sometimes, of course, there are several causes and factors influencing your snoring, for example, a deviated nasal septum plus weight gain, or a receding chin plus an allergy and a habitual drink at bedtime. So you and your doctor may need to direct treatment in several different directions.

The various treatments we will tell you about are targeted at all the potential causes of snoring. So the most important thing to do at the outset is to gather information about your particular snoring.

How Do You Know Whether You Snore?

You probably know you snore because someone who has slept with you or observed you during sleep has told you so. You have even stronger evidence if more than one person has told you, or if your regular bed-partner mentions it a lot.

Can you tell by yourself whether you snore? Some patients who come to the sleep disorders center at St. Michael's Hospital tell us, "I wake myself up with my snoring." However, occasionally waking up and realizing that you were snoring does not necessarily mean that your snoring is chronic or a problem. Your snoring may simply be an occasional thing.

In fact, for chronic snorers, it's usually just the opposite. Chronic snorers generally are not disturbed by their own snoring; they can sleep all night, never waking up, totally unaware of the noise they're making. At St. Michael's we asked 613 patients who had spent the night in the sleep lab to rate how much they thought they had snored that night as "none," "moderate," "severe," or "do not know." Of the 613 patients, 471 answered "do not know," and of the 75 patients who rated their snoring as "none," sleep recordings showed that only 29 were right. All the rest snored, some severely.

To determine your snoring facts, it's best to ask other people who might know, and to ask more than one person if possible, because your snoring may be perceived differently by different people. Some people are very sound sleepers and so may be totally undisturbed by their bed-partner's snoring, whereas others may wake up at the slightest sound, lie awake for hours, and finally be forced to go to a different room.

Sometimes even sleep technologists can disagree on the frequency and loudness of a person's snoring. Snoring sounds of 25 patients undergoing a sleep study were taped. When two technologists independently listened to the audiotape the next morning and counted the number of times each patient snored, they only agreed three out of four times.

Unrelated factors may also influence a person's perception of your snoring, sometimes subconsciously, without the person's realizing it. For example, if a couple is having marital difficulties, snoring may then assume major importance, and sometimes is claimed as the principal factor in breaking up the marriage. But when this is the case, there usually are other, deeper problems with the relationship.

The severity of snoring is often in the ears of the beholder. But if *several* or *many* people tell you that you snore loudly and frequently, you should believe them and investigate your snoring further.

Also remember that all noise is not necessarily snoring. You may have asthma or a respiratory infection or some other problem that causes noisy breathing when you sleep. Or you may make *both* noises: wheezing from asthma *plus* snoring.

Tape-Record Your Snoring

One way to know more about your snoring is to tape-record it. You can make a recording with an audiocassette recorder, using one that has the option of being voice activated, which will save tape. However, remember that usually on a voice-activated recording, the first part of sounds are often lost. You can also have your bedpartner make the recording, turning it on for typical samples of your snoring, especially when your snoring is worst and when there are episodes of stopped breathing.

Whichever method you use, be sure to have the microphone close to you. And if you intend to have your doctor listen to the tape, be sure to provide a good sample of what your snoring really sounds like. Often the first few attempts at taping do not truly reflect the loudness and frequency of a person's snoring. Be sure your bedpartner gets a good sample.

Making a video recording is even better. It can give the doctor a more complete picture of what your snoring is really like. It can also give strong clues to possible sleep apnea. On a video, in only a few minutes it can become apparent whether you have sleep apnea, and how significantly. Apnea usually follows a very characteristic sequence of events: First, there are a few breaths without any snoring at all, followed by breaths with progressively louder snoring. Then the snoring suddenly stops, with a few gasps or snorts, followed by a period of no breathing for ten seconds or more, which comes to an end with a very loud snort, sometimes waking up even the snorer. Then the person falls asleep again, and the same cycle of events repeats itself. During the absence of snoring, the sleeper appears to be gasping for breath, but unable to get any air into the lungs. The chest looks like it is "caving in" instead of rising up with each breath. A good video recording of you sleeping can be quite helpful in giving the doctor clues to the severity of your snoring and the possibility of sleep apnea.

It also helps if your bedpartner or helper can describe how your snoring varies in different ways, and if you have episodes of apnea, how long they lasted and how often they occurred. This sort of description can provide useful information to your doctor, as can answering the following questions:

- Does your snoring disturb people in the next room?
- Can it be heard two rooms away? on the other side of the house? downstairs? all the way to the neighbor's next door?
- Has your snoring become very much worse? Beginning when?

Note to spouses of snorers: If your snoring bedpartner refuses to believe that he (or she) snores or that his snoring could be a problem, tape-record his snoring and play the tape back to him. This should convince him that he does snore and that it is reasonable for you to be bothered, and—hopefully—it will even make him do something about it.

What Are Your Risk Factors?

If you suspect you snore, the first step to overcoming it is to determine whether you suffer from one of the three major risk factors connected to your lifestyle.

1. *Are you overweight?* People who are overweight are more likely than others to snore, and more likely to snore loudly and regularly. And if you snore and are overweight, you are more likely than someone of normal weight to have sleep apnea. At the St. Michael's sleep clinic, almost two-thirds of snorers with sleep apnea are significantly overweight, weighing on the average more than 50 percent over their ideal weight.

2. *Do you drink alcohol or take sleeping pills or tranquilizers before going to bed?* All of these actions can be a major factor in causing snoring or making it worse. And if you have sleep apnea, they can set up circumstances that can kill you. Don't forget that even one or two glasses of wine or beer, if consumed late in the evening, will aggravate snoring and apnea. You can change these lifestyle factors to help combat snoring and to decrease life-threatening apnea. In the next two chapters we will outline steps to help you do this.

3. *Do you smoke cigarettes?* You already know that smoking is bad for your health. Now you have another reason to become a non-smoker: smoking is a risk factor for snoring and apnea. We'll tell you of effective ways to become a nonsmoker in the next chapter.

Checking for Medical Causes

Aside from the big three lifestyle factors that can cause snoring, there are also many medical causes for snoring. This is one of the reasons you need to discuss your snoring with your physician. You should especially see your doctor if you have severe snoring that has just started recently and you haven't gained any weight. There is a chance it could be a tumor in the airway, an early sign of neuromuscular disease, or a hormonal problem.

All of the following medical problems have been implicated as possible causes of snoring. Your doctor might not think to ask about or check on these problems, so be sure to mention any such problems in your health background. Ask yourself the following questions:

Does your family have a history of heavy loud snoring? There seems to be a tendency to snoring in some families. If your father or mother were heavy loud snorers, it is more likely that you, too, will be a snorer.

Do you have a short thick neck? a receding chin? Persons with these characteristics are more likely to snore, and if they snore they are more likely to have apnea. At St. Michael's almost 20 percent of men and women with apnea had a collar size greater than 18, compared to only 4 percent of snorers without sleep apnea.

Do you have a broken nose? a deviated septum? nasal obstruction due to a chronic allergy or infection? Any of these could cause nasal obstruction and increased nasal resistance, making you breathe through your mouth and thus increasing your likelihood of both snoring and apnea. Also if you wake up in the morning, or sometimes even in the middle of the night, needing a drink of water because of a dry mouth, this is a sign that you are probably a mouth breather—another indication of nasal obstruction and increased nasal resistance.

Do you have thyroid problems? Hypothyroidism is often a cause of apnea. Thyroid hormone replacement treatment has been shown to reverse apnea in most cases when a person has low thyroid.

Do you have asthma? Asthma is sometimes associated with snoring and apnea. Often treating asthma will help snoring, and conversely, treating apnea will often relieve asthma.

Are you taking any medications? We've already mentioned sleeping pills and tranquilizers, which can make snoring and apnea worse. But some other medicines can sometimes cause problems, too. For example, sometimes aspirin, oral contraceptives, and estrogens can bring about endocrine changes that cause nasal congestion. Decongestant nasal drops and sprays may work for a while, but they can rebound and actually make congestion worse. Some drugs used to treat high blood pressure can lead to chronic nasal congestion. Talk to your doctor about medications you are taking and whether any of them might be causing a side effect such as nasal congestion, central nervous system depression, or muscle relaxation that could be affecting your snoring. But absolutely do not change medications without discussing with your doctor possible changes and the potential consequences.

Check Your Throat

Dr. Takenosuke Ikematsu studied an astounding 25,000 snorers from 1952 to 1991 in his practice in Japan, measuring the internal dimensions of the throats of his patients and correlating the measurements with degrees of snoring. He found that more than 90 percent of snorers showed one or more of the following throat conditions: elongated or enlarged uvula, drooping soft palate, large prominent tonsils, narrowing of the back of the throat, or a large tongue.

You can check yourself for some of these conditions. Stand in front of a mirror, open your mouth wide, and look inside. A snorer's mouth tends to look crowded and small. Here are the things to check for: a large bulky tongue that takes up lots of space in the mouth; a bulky soft palate that takes up room at the top of your throat; a uvula (the little piece of tissue hanging from the roof of the mouth in the back) that is large and inflamed because it is constantly bouncing against the walls of the throat during recurring snoring vibrations and closures; and large tonsils in the back of the throat. All of these anatomical features with these characteristics take up space in your throat, making the airway smaller. This increases airway resistance, causing further collapse and vibrations of the tissues, creating loud noise. Also studies show that snorers with floppy and small throats are more likely to have sleep apnea.

If you have any of these problems or other problems such as a broken nose, you probably need to see an ear, nose, and throat (ENT) specialist for an evaluation of your condition.

Other Things to Tell Your Doctor

We believe as part of every check-up physicians should ask patients if they snore, have stopped breathing when sleeping, or have other sleep problems. But if your doctor doesn't ask, you should tell him on your own. In order for your doctor to accurately analyze your snoring problem, you'll need to be prepared to answer these questions:

Do you only snore on your back or in any position? Some people only need a nudge to turn over and stop snoring. For others it makes no difference. If you only snore when you're on your back, it's called "positional snoring." There are a number of things you can do to help keep you from sleeping on your back. We'll talk in chapter 8 about the things that happen when you sleep on your back, and we'll give you some simple things to do to help prevent this kind of snoring.

Do you snore on most nights, or only under certain circumstances? Tell your doctor if you only snore on nights when you have had alcohol or have taken an antihistamine, tranquilizer, or sleeping pill, or if snoring occurs more often when you are overly tired or have a cold.

When and under what circumstances did your snoring start? Did it start when you gained weight, or when you started or stopped a medication? Did it develop gradually or start suddenly? Knowing this will help your doctor pinpoint treatments. For example, if you snore during allergy season, an allergy to pollen is likely the cause, and snoring may be relieved with treatment of the allergy.

How bad is your snoring? Does it keep just your bedpartner awake or everyone in the house?

Do you snort, gasp, or stop breathing? How frequently? These are the main signs of sleep apnea, and if they occur frequently during the night, you need treatment.

Do you have headaches in the morning? feel irritable? depressed? find it difficult to interact with other people? have trouble concentrating? feel more tired than you think you should? Has your sex drive decreased? These can all be the result of fragmented sleep or your not getting enough oxygen in your blood at night because of snoring or apnea.

Are you impotent? This is a symptom sometimes associated with apnea. A study in a sleep lab can be designed to detect whether you have erections during sleep and thus help identify whether your impotence is psychological or physical and perhaps related to apnea.

Are you restless at night, kicking your legs and arms? Some people move their arms and legs so much that they wear holes in their sheets. This restless activity is frequently associated with sleep apnea, and in many patients, treatment of the sleep apnea will eliminate the leg kicks.

Do you grind your teeth at night? Tooth grinding, called *bruxism*, is not associated with snoring or apnea, but it can cause problems, including severe headache and jaw pain on awakening. Talk to your dentist. Dentists prescribe 3.5 million protective nightguards a year for this problem. If the problem is severe, you may also choose to have a sleep study to see whether there are other sleep problems involved.

Keep a Snoring Log

Some people find it helpful to keep a "snoring log." To do this, have your bedpartner keep track of your snoring over several different nights and under different conditions, carefully noting down your rate and loudness of snoring and the number of episodes of apnea, if any. Then you can compare the severity of your snoring at different times to see if there is a correlation to circumstances such as whether you do or do not drink in the evening, or do or do not take a sleeping pill, or whether there is a difference when you have gained or lost weight.

Just remember, it should be your bedpartner who keeps the log, not you, because snorers are usually unaware of their snoring.

If you go to a sleep disorders center or a sleep laboratory for any problem, it is almost certain that you will be asked to fill out a questionnaire dealing with your sleeping habits, snoring patterns, and daytime functioning. You will also be given a sleep diary to fill out at home, usually for two weeks, describing your sleep habits (what time you go to bed, what time you turn the lights out, if you snack or drink and when, what time you wake, etc.). By analyzing your replies to the questionnaire and studying your sleep diary, your doctor will be able to determine the possible nighttime problems that might be causing your poor daytime functioning and vice versa.

And remember, don't worry if you have just a few apnea episodes. We'll tell you later in this chapter how many episodes should be a matter of concern.

Evaluating Morning Fatigue

Feeling tired in the morning, not refreshed by sleep, or even feeling worse than you did in the evening before you went to bed is a symptom that should always make you seek medical advice. Obviously we are referring to being tired in the morning on a regular basis, not just because you stayed up late last night partying or writing an overdue report. Chronic morning tiredness could be due to snoring, apnea, or other medical causes.

People with sleep apnea, for example, have a very fragmented sleep, constantly interrupted by brain wave arousals that occur at the termination of each apnea episode. As a result, they do not have refreshing sleep and get up in the morning frequently feeling worse or the same as they did in the evening before they went to bed. During the day they continue to feel tired, have difficulty concentrating, and complain about poor memory, lack of energy, and generally poor functioning.

Snorers and patients with sleep apnea both frequently have morning headache as well as tiredness. There are questionnaires which you will fill out in the sleep clinic that allow your doctors to assess your tiredness.

Evaluating Excessive Daytime Sleepiness

Is sleepiness during the day a problem for you? One of the most important symptoms suggestive of snoring and sleep apnea, and also one that is difficult to assess and quantify, is excessive daytime sleepiness. What does it mean to feel *excessively* sleepy during the day? Does it mean falling asleep when reading a book, watching television, or sitting quietly, such as after eating lunch, in a boring lecture, or in the theater? If you only get sleepy occasionally, or only when you're especially tired, it's probably not what would be classified as excessive daytime sleepiness. But if you feel drowsy most of the time, or you doze off while driving a car, operating machinery, attending important meetings, or talking, or if you feel sleepy at other times when you don't want to, it probably *is* excessive daytime sleepiness, and should be a matter of concern. If you often feel exhausted during the day, if sleepiness often interferes with your work or your social life, or if sleepiness has ever caused you to have an accident or near accident while driving a car, operating machinery, or doing anything else, it should be a matter of concern.

Many snorers with apnea have become so used to their poor daytime functioning that they consider it normal and do not complain about it to their doctors. When their sleep apnea is diagnosed and treated, they are generally amazed at how much better they function.

An actuary who worked for an insurance company came into the clinic at St. Michael's one day because of snoring. He denied feeling bad or being sleepy or tired. But a sleep study showed that he had severe sleep apnea. Treatment was recommended and with some reluctance he said he would try it. After three days he called to say how surprised he was to feel markedly refreshed during the day and that his productivity had increased dramatically. Being an actuary, he estimated that his income would go up by $35,000 per year because he now was more efficient and could work longer hours. After one year, when he came in for a reassessment, he said that he never expected that he would feel so well, and in fact his income had gone up by $50,000.

There are tests designed to evaluate how sleepy you are during the day and distinguish this from daytime tiredness. Some are questionnaires to assess daytime sleepiness. Two are objective tests done in the sleep lab—the maintenance of wakefulness test (MWT) and the multiple sleep latency test (MSLT). The most common test is the MSLT, which scientifically assesses how sleepy you are. The test is done in the sleep lab on the day following a night of sleeping in the lab. During the day you are asked to lie down every two hours for twenty minutes, and technicians measure whether and how fast you fall asleep. An average person might fall asleep once, usually after lunch. A person with excessive sleepiness might fall asleep at several or all of the tests. You can do an at-home version: After a normal night's sleep, lie down every two hours throughout the next day, say at 9 A.M., 11 A.M., 1 P.M., and 3 P.M. Each time hold a set of keys between two fingers over the side of the bed or sofa when you lie down. When you fall asleep, the keys will drop, and the noise will wake you up. Have a clock in view. If the keys drop in less than five minutes or you fall asleep at more than one test, you probably have excessive daytime sleepiness. Try getting two hours more sleep each night for the next week (some people are sleepy in the day simply because they aren't getting enough sleep), then try the tests again. If you are still excessively sleepy, you should seek help at a sleep disorders center.

Be sure to tell the clinic whether you are taking any medications, including over-the-counter ones, or whether you have made any recent changes in medications. Certain medications, as well as street drugs, can cause excessive daytime sleepiness. Or sleepiness can be caused by starting or stopping a medication or changing the dosage.

Being excessively sleepy is not natural and you should not have to suffer with the bad feeling and poor functioning that it causes. It's possible you simply are not allowing yourself to get enough sleep, but it's also possible that nighttime sleep disorders are causing daytime problems. In addition to snoring and apnea, or simply insufficient sleep, you might have asthma that repeatedly awakens you at night, or you might have a condition called *narcolepsy* that causes you to fall asleep during the day, or your legs might twitch during sleep and repeatedly awaken you. Diabetes, anemia, hypothyroidism, congestive heart failure, kidney disease, depression, shift work changes, and pregnancy can all interfere with restful sleep and cause fatigue and sleepiness during the day.

The important thing to remember is that people have often been called lazy or stupid, perhaps even ridiculed because of their problem of sleepiness, but the truth is that excessive daytime sleepiness is almost never caused by a psychiatric or psychological problem, but rather is usually caused by a medical condition such as apnea or some other correctable problem. Sometimes people may think they have insomnia because they wake up so often at night for unknown reasons, but often that unknown reason is sleep apnea. If your doctor mistakenly thinks you have insomnia and prescribes sleeping pills "to help you sleep better" or tranquilizers "to calm you down," it's a dangerous fix. These drugs depress respiration, and if your nonbreathing episodes are already long or frequent, such drugs can make them worse enough to kill you.

When Testing at Home Isn't Conclusive

Final determination of the causes of your excessive daytime sleepiness and other symptoms of sleep disorders can only be done with a sleep study. But many patients are reluctant to go to a sleep lab. They worry that because of sleeping in strange surroundings, in a different bed, with monitoring equipment, and with strangers watching, they will be uncomfortable and that their sleep and snoring will not be representative of what happens at home.

Is there a difference in snoring from night to night, or a difference in sleeping at home or in a sleep lab? Sleep researcher Dr. Frèdèric Sériès and colleagues of Quebec, Canada, studied fourteen snorers to check out this problem. They measured their snoring on three occasions during a two-week period, with two sleep tests done at home and one in the sleep lab. They found two interesting things. First, snoring frequency measured on the two nights at home was almost identical to the snoring frequency measured in the laboratory. Second, snoring loudness, contrary to what you might expect, was greater in the laboratory than at home. Perhaps the reason is that in the laboratory you would sleep more on your back than on your side because it's harder to turn over on your side when you're attached to all the monitoring equipment. Therefore, you do not need to worry that findings in the sleep lab will not be representative of what happens at home in your own bed.

If the laboratory sleep study does not demonstrate that snoring or other sleep disorders are causing your problems, and if your bedpartner or family still insists that your snoring keeps everybody awake, your doctor will most likely disregard the lab findings and will offer you some treatment options to try on a trial basis. It is also important to have lab studies to determine whether you have apnea or another condition that could cause noisy breathing; you might be treating one when you really have the other. The sleep lab will also check for the possibility of narcolepsy, which also can cause excessive daytime sleepiness. However, narcolepsy is different from sleep apnea in many respects: People with narcolepsy may exhibit sleep paralysis, a feeling of being unable to move their limbs as they are falling asleep or waking up. People with narcolepsy also have hallucinations, and many sometimes have sudden urges to sleep so that they just fall down, losing all muscle tone. In severe cases of narcolepsy, the person may have a sleep attack when excited or may actually fall asleep in the middle of talking, eating, or making love. Your doctor should also check for anemia, which can cause daytime fatigue but is not associated with snoring.

There are many questionnaires that have been designed to determine the presence of excessive daytime sleepiness. But one problem is that some of them are very lengthy, and most of the answers reflect your own, or your bedpartner's, subjective assessment of how you feel and act during the day. You or your mate may exaggerate the feeling or underestimate it, or you may feel very tired during the day, not because of sleep apnea, but because of other reasons.

One of the more common questionnaires used to assess daytime sleepiness in sleep laboratories is the Epworth sleepiness scale (ESS), which consists of eight questions, all describing certain situations and asking you how likely you are to fall asleep in these situations. If you go to a sleep disorders center, it is very likely that you will be asked to fill out such a questionnaire.

Considering the many causes of excessive daytime sleepiness, don't be disappointed if a sleep study shows that your daytime tiredness is not caused by sleep apnea. Be happy that this condition has been ruled out, and look, with your doctor, for another possible reason.

A Sleep Apnea Quiz

How can you tell whether you have sleep apnea? Answer these questions:

1. Are you a loud habitual snorer?
2. Do you feel tired and groggy on waking?
3. Are you often sleepy during the day?
4. Have you been observed to choke, snort, gasp, or hold your breath during sleep?

If you answered yes to any of these questions, you could have sleep apnea. You should discuss the symptoms with your physician or a sleep specialist.

If you don't have any of these symptoms, but you think others you know might have sleep apnea, you should give each of them a copy of this book and encourage them to see a physician. It could change or even save their lives.

Home Monitoring Equipment

If you are really worried about going to a sleep laboratory and not being able to fall asleep, you may ask your doctor if it is possible to monitor your sleep at home. You cannot set it up by yourself; it has to be done by an experienced person, and the results have to be scored by a sleep technologist and interpreted by a physician. Some systems require a technologist to come to your home, set up the equipment, demonstrate how it works, and show you how to put on various monitors and start and stop the equipment. Other systems can be demonstrated to you during a clinic visit in the afternoon and you yourself will attach the monitoring apparatus when you go to bed. If you need to get up in the middle of the night to go to the bathroom, you will know how to disconnect the equipment and how to reattach it when you come back to bed. The portable monitor records data all night, storing the recorded data in the computer memory or on a disk. The data can be downloaded and analyzed at a central laboratory the following day.

Monitoring at home is not as complete and informative as having the tests and recordings done in a sleep lab, but the advantage is that it costs considerably less.

Most varieties of home monitoring equipment are capable of recording breathing efforts, airflow, blood oxygen levels, heart rate, snoring patterns, and body positions. Some, but not all, can also record brain waves, muscle twitches, and eye movements during sleep.

The disadvantage of home monitoring methods is that there haven't been any large-scale validation studies comparing the results obtained using home monitoring equipment with those obtained in the sleep laboratory. Also it is difficult to record stages of sleep using home monitors; in fact, with some home monitors it may be difficult to distinguish between sleep and wakefulness. Nevertheless, the use of in-home sleep studies is growing because they cost less, and as development continues, this method will become more sophisticated and reliable.

What's Your Snore Score? What Did You Find? What Should You Do?

If after performing any of the snoring tests in this chapter you found anything that might be causing your snoring or influencing your risk of snoring or of developing apnea, consider your finding a call for action. If what you found is a lifestyle factor such as being overweight, taking sleeping pills, or drinking alcohol before going to bed, you should begin a program to change that. If what you found is a medical condition or an anatomical condition, then you should call your doctor to talk about it. Don't wait until your next checkup.

For people who have heart trouble, snoring and sleep apnea can make their condition worse because of the reduced oxygen levels. If you have heart disease and if chest pain wakes you from sleep, it may indicate sleep apnea. This is something you should discuss with your doctor as soon as you can.

An occasional episode of apnea is quite common and is not significant. However, if you have severe snoring or signs of significant apnea—more than ten to fifteen episodes per hour of sleep—then you should seek medical help. Make notes of the things you have discovered from the testing you did, and discuss your findings with your doctor. Also be sure to tell your doctor how much alcohol you use, whether you take sleeping pills, tranquilizers, or muscle relaxants, and whether you smoke. If you made an audio or video recording, take this with you to the doctor also.

Most snorers, especially those with mild snoring, do not have sleep apnea. But there is some concern that years of snoring may cause damage to tissues in the throat, which can increase the risk of developing sleep apnea in the future. Because of this, and because your health stands to benefit from help, we urge you to read what we have learned about the latest treatments being used in world-renowned sleep disorders centers and apply them to your own snoring situation. You will sleep better, you will be healthier, and you will feel less tired during the day. Your bedpartner and others suffering from secondhand snoring will be better off, too.

4

Snoring, Smoking, and Drinking

There are several lifestyle habits that are the most important risk factors in snoring: being overweight, taking sleeping pills and muscle relaxants, drinking alcohol before going to bed, and smoking. We will talk about how to deal with being overweight and taking pills later on. For now, let's deal with the latter two factors—smoking and alcohol.

It's logical that these two habits contribute to snoring—we all know that cigarette smoke can irritate the membranes of the nose and throat, and you've probably observed that alcohol before bedtime can cause snoring in a person who ordinarily does not snore, or worsen snoring in someone who is already a snorer. Now epidemiological studies consistently have proven scientifically the association with snoring.

The Evidence

One of the first studies that linked smoking and alcohol to snoring took place in 1988 when Dr. John Bloom and his colleagues at the University of Arizona College of Medicine in Tucson asked more than 2,000 people about their snoring and found that there were more snorers among smokers than among nonsmokers. In women who smoked, the prevalence of snoring was four times higher than in nonsmokers; in men who smoked, the prevalence of snoring was two and a half times higher than in nonsmokers. Furthermore, the more cigarettes people smoked, the higher their risk of snoring. If the smokers were also obese, the snoring prevalence went up even more. Even ex-smokers were more at risk of snoring than those who never smoked. However, the researchers found that after four years of not smoking, the ex-smokers' snoring dropped to that of the never-smokers, which may explain why several years of nonsmoking may be necessary to eliminate snoring.

The Tucson researchers also found that among people who drank alcohol before going to sleep, there was a high prevalence of snoring, much higher than in those who did *not* use alcohol at night.

Then in 1994 Dr. David Wetter and a team of researchers from the University of Wisconsin in Madison reported on a study of more than 800 students at the university. They not only asked these people about their smoking and snoring, but actually carried out sleep studies with them. It was found that current smokers were more than two times higher at risk of snoring than never-smokers. Those who smoked more than forty cigarettes per day were three times more at risk of snoring and forty times more at risk of significant sleep apnea than those who never smoked. Also, ex-smokers were more at risk of snoring and sleep apnea when compared to never-smokers.

Other research showed that alcohol could cause apnea in snorers, and in those who already had apnea, alcohol made it much worse.

We know how difficult it is to make serious lifestyle changes, but if you do, you will be taking one step in your fight against snoring.

Although obesity and alcohol are both more important than smoking as risk factors in snoring, we are beginning with smoking because it has so many other ill effects on your health and well-being.

Cigarettes and Snoring

If you're already a nonsmoker, you have already mastered the first step in your no-snoring program. Smoking can ruin your health, cause early death—and along the way, mess up your sleep.

If you're still a smoker and need motivation, consider these facts: Smokers have a higher death rate from heart disease, stroke, and cancer. Smoking is by far the major cause of chronic bronchitis, emphysema, and lung cancer. As a smoker, you have more shortness of breath, more ulcers, and more kidney disease than nonsmokers. Smoking can decrease your visual perception, increase your serum cholesterol and triglycerides, and aggravate your allergies. It can decrease sex drive and response, cause infertility or birth problems, and cause premature deliveries or birth defects. Smoking can cause skin to wrinkle and aggravate dental problems. If you're a woman who smokes and uses birth control pills, you have a greater chance of stroke or heart attack. Nicotine increases your heart rate and blood pressure, narrows blood vessels, increases the tendency of the blood to clot, and slows down peripheral circulation. And smoking makes your hair, clothes, and breath smell bad. It is estimated that smoking causes about 450,000 premature deaths per year in the United States, with an average loss of life of about seven years. Another way to look at it: tobacco use leads to death in one of every five otherwise healthy people. Another sobering estimate: by the year 2020 about 10 million people world-wide will die *each year* from smoking. Total cost in medical and hospital bills, lost wages, and reduced productivity for just one country is in the billions.

How Cigarettes Increase Risk of Snoring

Cigarette smoking irritates upper airways and causes them to become inflamed. This inflammation affects the entire length of the airway— from the throat to the smallest bronchi leading to the lungs. Inflamed airways are narrow and have poor muscle tone, and so are more sus-ceptible to further narrowing and collapse when you lie down on your back and go to sleep. Breathing through a narrow and floppy airway causes the walls of the airway to vibrate, which manifests as snoring. Sometimes the airway narrows so much that it actually closes, resulting in obstructive apnea.

Cigarettes Can Also Cause Insomnia and Other Sleep Disturbances

Smoking is associated not only with snoring, but also with many other sleep disturbances. For example, Drs. David Wetter and Terry Young of the University of Wisconsin found after asking 3,516 people about their sleep and smoking habits that difficulties in getting to sleep and com-plaints about nonrestorative sleep were more than double among smokers than among nonsmokers. Similarly, Drs. Barbara Phillips and Frederick Danner of the University of Kentucky in Lexington found af-ter interviewing 484 people (99 of whom were high school students) that the cigarette smokers had significantly more problems with going to sleep, staying asleep, daytime sleepiness, minor accidents, and de-pression.

Insomnia is one of the major things that most smokers complain about. Nicotine keeps people awake. It's a stimulant, just as caffeine is. In fact, it has been shown that cigarettes not only raise blood pressure and speed heart rate but also stimulate brain wave activity. Some smokers may also wake up in the middle of the night because their bodies are experiencing withdrawal symptoms.

Experiments by Dr. Anthony Kales and a team of scientists at Pennsylvania State University showed that when a group of men who had smoked from one to three packs of cigarettes a day stopped smoking, they fell asleep faster and woke less during the night.

So if you're a smoker, becoming a nonsmoker might well help your snoring *and* your insomnia.

Choose Your Plan for Becoming a Nonsmoker

The government's first antismoking report was published in the United States in 1964. From then until now, the percentage of smokers in the population has dropped tremendously. It appears that two out of three people who had smoked at one time have now stopped. You can, too. Not only will it be a positive step toward less snoring and better health, but you will *feel* better and it will give you a new feeling of control over your life.

The team at St. Michael's Hospital recognizes that smoking is an important risk factor in snoring; consequently, in each patient we take a careful smoking history, stress the importance of becoming a nonsmoker, and advise smokers to attend a smoking cessation program.

You can choose to get rid of cigarettes gradually or cold turkey. If you choose to stop gradually, first chart your smoking habits by recording each cigarette you smoke and under what circumstances, and rating how much you need it. Then on day one, eliminate the cigarettes you need the least. On day three or four, eliminate half of the cigarettes you need a little. A day or two later, eliminate the rest of the in-between cigarettes. At the beginning of the second week, attack the cigarettes that you need the most by smoking only half a cigarette at each of the I-need-it-most times. Every day eliminate one of these half cigarettes, keeping your chart with you so that you don't backslide into smoking any of those you have gotten rid of. By the end of the third week, you should be down to a single half cigarette. Smoke it, and flush it. And never go back.

Most studies show, however, it is best to choose a specific date and quit cold turkey. Some people force themselves to smoke as many cigarettes as they can the day before they start their plan, to build up an aversion to the cigarettes. (Don't do this if you have cardiovascular or lung disease.)

Whichever method you choose, in order to become a nonsmoker you need to overcome both of the two major factors responsible for your smoking: nicotine addiction and the *habit* of smoking.

Think about what habits may be trapping you into smoking. What are the circumstances under which you often automatically light up? Do you usually light up a cigarette when you drive, when you have a cup of coffee or a drink, when you go to the bathroom, or when you talk on the telephone? Try "pack tracking" for a week, writing down each and every time you light a cigarette and under what circumstances. Stick a notebook in the pocket where you keep your cigarettes, or wrap a pencil and paper around the pack with a rubber band. You may be surprised at how many times you automatically light up from habit without thinking. These are the times to especially watch out for. Try substitutions: When you want a cigarette, drink a glass of water, get up from your desk and take a short walk or do some exercises, have a low-calorie snack, or have tea, hot chocolate, or a fruit drink instead. If you smoked first thing in the morning, get up and do some exercises instead, or jump immediately into the shower. If you always smoked after a meal, get up from the table immediately and clear the dishes or go for a walk. If you smoked when you were around other people who smoked, then for several weeks avoid those people and spend your time with nonsmoking friends and in nonsmoking places.

Stay Motivated

The next big thing to make your nonsmoking plan successful is to be seriously motivated.

Make a list of reasons why you want to be a nonsmoker, and look at it every day: fewer wrinkles, less chance of having lung or heart disease or cancer, less dental work, better-smelling clothes and hair, better sex. Put a big jar on your dresser or desk, and every day put in the money you would have spent on cigarettes. Visit the dentist and have your teeth cleaned so you'll want to keep them that way. The motivating trigger for some people is to have their lung function measured in the doctor's office and learn that their "lung age" is twenty years more than their regular age.

Some Things That Will Help

Smoking is an addiction, and therefore the smoker who is willing to overcome the addiction usually requires much support. Some patients are capable of doing it alone, but these are few. Most smokers need a structured program that provides them with information, positive reinforcement of their decision to quit smoking, and group support from their peers undergoing the same difficult withdrawal. So whether you choose to stop smoking gradually or cold turkey, bear in mind that all the many studies done on smoking cessation show that there is a higher success rate if you use one or more methods of support. It can be as simple as having a buddy who also is eager to become a nonsmoker. Some people have found relaxation exercises, group workshops, acupuncture, or hypnosis helpful for an extra benefit system. You may want to consult with your physician, a psychologist, or other therapist, and try a stop-smoking program or group workshop recommended by them. Many hospitals have smoking cessation clinics that provide group sessions, motivational information, and tips on nutrition to avoid gaining weight—a common fear of many smokers. Some lung associations also have excellent smoking cessation programs. Think about which supports will work best for you and check them out.

Many people also find it helpful to use nicotine chewing gum or nicotine skin patches, which help by temporarily replacing some of the nicotine that cigarettes would supply. One brand has additional medication on the patch that helps some people stay calm and control cravings during the withdrawal period. Both the gum and the patches come in different strengths. Also on the market now are nicotine inhalers and nicotine nasal sprays. If you choose to use nicotine replacement methods, see your doctor because you should not use this method if you have heart problems, have recently had a stroke, or have an allergy to nicotine. Nor should you use them if you are pregnant or breastfeeding or have certain skin disorders. *Do not smoke when using nicotine gum or the patch!* It can severely overdose you on nicotine and cause such side effects as severe headaches, vomiting, blurred vision, fainting, and other symptoms.

People who use nicotine gum to help stop smoking usually chew

---

THE FOUR D'S

The American Lung Association has put together a plan called the "Four D's." Whenever you feel the urge for a cigarette, try the four D's:

1. Delay. The urge to smoke will pass whether you smoke or not. By delaying the cigarette for, say, thirty minutes or even fifteen, you will have taken control instead of the cigarette addiction controlling you.

2. Deep-breathe. Take ten deep breaths instead of a cigarette break. It will help you relax.

3. Drink a lot of water. It counteracts the urge to smoke and helps clear your system.

4. Do something different. Only a few minutes of substitute activity are needed. Take a shower, wash your hands, do the dishes—it's hard to keep a cigarette lit around water. Brush your teeth or suck a mint for a clean-mouth taste. Exercise, walk, water the plants, make love, dance to your favorite music, iron a shirt—whatever it takes.

---

ten to fifteen pieces a day. Each piece is chewed slowly so that the nicotine is absorbed through the lining of the mouth (not by swallowing it).

Nicotine patches are most helpful for smokers of more than twenty cigarettes per day. The patch is applied to the hip, back, shoulder, or upper arm on skin that is clean and dry and free of creams or powder. You wear it for twenty-four hours and put a new one in a different location each time you use it. Usually you use strong dosage patches for several weeks, then lighter strength patches, until you can go without any nicotine at all. If you have any side effects such as headache, insomnia, abnormal dreams, dizziness, or stomach upset, contact your doctor so that the dosage may be adjusted. Some people experience tingling of the skin under the patch, but this usually disappears within a few hours.

Others who are trying to kick the habit find it helpful to take low doses of an antidepressant. A study of smokers at sixteen cities in the United States found that a low dose of Prozac (30 milligrams) taken every day for ten weeks helped them stay off cigarettes. Reports also started coming in from patients taking another antidepressant, Wellbutrin, that was helping them lose their desire to smoke. So doctors started trying the drug for smoking cessation. In late 1997 a nonsmoking version of Wellbutrin, named Zyban, became available for use. How well does it work? Of some 2,600 smokers who took part in a ten-week study, 58 percent of those who used both Zyban and a nicotine patch kicked their cigarette habit. That was compared to 49 percent who used Zyban alone and 36 percent who used the patch alone. Zyban tablets are taken for a week before you stop smoking, then for seven to twelve weeks, sometimes longer. Side effects are rare, but can include a dry sensation in the mouth and insomnia.

Doctors believe Zyban helps smokers in two ways. First, it stimulates the release of dopamine, a pleasure-inducing brain chemical, the same one that nicotine is believed to trigger. Second, the drug seems to take the edge off anxiety and irritability that smokers sometimes feel when they're trying to quit. As one former smoker who became a nonsmoker by using the drug said: "It takes care of the times when something stressful happens—your boss yells at you, you got wrongly billed again by the telephone company and can't reach a real person to credit your account—times when you would ordinarily reach for a cigarette, but the pill takes that edge off and you don't need the cigarette." But remember, Zyban and Prozac are drugs. Discuss their use with your doctor.

A number of other drugs, including other patch medicines, are in the developmental stage, and many are undergoing clinical trials at this time.

More important than drugs is your determination and the psychological support from others. Whether you choose to join an organized group, find a buddy who also wants to be a nonsmoker, or do it alone, it's important in the early stages of building the no-smoking habit to stay away from other smokers and smoke-filled environments. Stay away from smoky bars, and eat in the nonsmoking section of restaurants. Surrounding yourself with a nonsmoking culture will make it easier for you to hold on to your resolve to be free of smoking.

In addition, most people find that taking a strong vitamin-mineral supplement rich in vitamin C, B vitamins, calcium, and magnesium will help fight stress and replace the vitamins that have been destroyed by smoking. Also keep on hand a good supply of fruit juice, chewing gum, carrots, celery, popcorn, nuts, and other sugar-free snacks to chew on. Drink large amounts of water, even as often as every hour, to help flush the nicotine out of your system. When you crave a cigarette, substitute a walk, swim, bike ride, or other exercise to help work out the tension, or chew on your carrots and celery sticks. Get plenty of sleep so that you are well rested and can more easily remain in control all day. Some people have found it helpful to use a combination of Chinese herbs to counteract some of the withdrawal symptoms. Herbs that have been shown to have a calming effect are *Acorus* and *Polygala tenuifolia.* Herbs that help moisturize the lungs and counteract cough are *Codonopsis* (dang shen), *Adenophora, Ophiopogon, Glehnia, Houttuynia herba,* and *Plantago.* All are available in health food stores, often in combination.

It is natural to temporarily have withdrawal symptoms as you get away from the nicotine. You may (or may not) experience dizziness, fatigue, irritability, restlessness, emotional outbursts, lack of concentration, sleep disturbances, tremors, headache, increased appetite, or just plain craving. For most people it takes about twelve weeks to be totally comfortable. Keep reminding yourself that withdrawal symptoms are temporary and *will* disappear.

Rewards

The last day as a smoker, throw away all remaining cigarettes and your ashtrays and lighters. Check yourself out and say to yourself, "I am a nonsmoker, and I'm looking good!"

At the end of your first day without one dirty cigarette, reward yourself. Spend the money you have saved from not buying cigarettes. Find someone to share your joy at being smoke-free and go out and celebrate!

If you do have a cigarette after you quit, don't be hard on yourself. Just get back on the program. You've learned so much, it will be easier this time.

Some people don't want to stop smoking or want to return to it because they haven't found sufficient rewards. They say, "It's one of the few pleasures I have." But if being a nonsmoker solves your snoring problem, then taking that last puff can mean more than saying good-bye to the bad, it can also mean saying hello to snoring less, sleeping better, and feeling better the next day.

There are no magic bullets that will permit you to quit smoking without effort. Nicotine gum or patches, self-locking cigarette cases that can only be opened at specific times, and other devices are simply aids that can only be effective when combined with your determination to quit. There is no single best method to quit smoking that will fit everyone. You will get the best results from educating yourself about the dangers of smoking, getting ongoing moral and physical support from professionals, friends, and family members, and going to group sessions to discuss the temptations to restart smoking and how to deal with them.

The Good News

Besides feeling better, being healthier, coughing less, and snoring less, if you are taking any kind of medication, you may be able to lower the dosage because being a nonsmoker will improve your health so much. Stay in touch with your doctor and follow the advice given.

Social attitudes toward smoking have changed a lot in the last few years, especially since the disclosures that the tobacco companies have lied and manipulated people to become addicted—a fact that most smokers know. By becoming a nonsmoker, you will have rid yourself of their control. You will have taken charge.

The other good news is the money you will have saved. How much do you pay for a pack of cigarettes? How many packs do you smoke in a year? Multiply it out and see what you will save!

Protect Your Rights against Secondhand Smoke

Just recently, the AMA reported even more new evidence of the serious medical effects of secondhand smoke. Even after you quit smoking, you definitely can still be affected by somebody else's smoking. The rights of nonsmokers are being more and more respected as more people join the ranks of nonsmokers. Many countries also are passing laws that prohibit smoking in public places and workplaces.

If someone asks your permission to smoke, stand up for your rights: smile pleasantly and say, "Thank you so much for asking—I would really appreciate it if you do not smoke." And if someone lights up in a no-smoking area, feel free to report it to the airplane flight attendant or the restaurant manager, who will probably be more than willing to remedy the situation.

If It's Your Spouse Who Smokes and Snores

There are ways in which you can help others to change.

First, don't nag. You can't make someone stop smoking. Smokers must make their own decisions. The desire for change must come from within. You can help most by being genuinely concerned and supportive. Ask the smoker what you could do that would be most helpful. If he (or she) says to leave him alone, then give him space. Just let him know you admire him for his self-determination. Be there to give positive reinforcement when it's appropriate or requested.

If your spouse wants to stop smoking, but talks about the deep craving, you might mention that the craving is supposed to last only three and a half minutes, then decreases. Dance a waltz together, go for a walk, take a shower together, have a pillow fight, tell jokes—take turns finding something interesting to do for three and a half minutes.

Alcohol and Snoring

There was a story in Ann Landers' column about a woman married twenty-four years to a man who snored. "His snoring under ordinary circumstances is enough to shake the fixtures," the woman wrote, "but when he has had a few drinks, he makes such a racket, the people in the upstairs apartment bang on the floor with what must be a sledgehammer." When they went on an overnight train, the people in the next compartment knocked on the door and asked if she could do something to quiet her husband. "Yes," she said, "but it's against the law."

The role of alcohol in snoring is one of the first things the staff at our sleep clinic discuss with patients who come to St. Michael's with snoring problems. Alcohol is a very important risk factor.

A single alcoholic drink before bedtime can cause snoring in a person who ordinarily does not snore, or can worsen snoring in someone who is already a snorer. Or it can result in obstructive sleep apnea condition and its dangers, especially if the person is also overweight.

One case especially showed how strong the influence of alcohol can be on snoring. A 37-year-old man was referred to the sleep laboratory at St. Michael's for investigation of his nighttime seizures. He was not a snorer—his wife never commented or complained about any snoring. There was nothing in his history to suggest sleep apnea. Everyone was totally surprised at the results of his sleep study. The recordings showed that he snored loudly and frequently throughout the night, and he had rather severe apnea. When asked if there was anything different about his actions during the day before his sleep study, he said that he had been very apprehensive about the sleep study. He had arrived early at the laboratory, and rather than wait, he decided to visit one of the local drinking establishments. (The hospital is located right in the middle of downtown Toronto and there is no shortage of bars in the area.) He had one scotch and one beer, and then, much less apprehensive, came back to the laboratory. Within less than two hours, he was in bed with all of the equipment in place, sound asleep and snoring loudly. The sleep study was repeated the next night, after he was warned not to drink any alcohol. His snoring was minimal and his stopped-breathing episodes were well within normal limits. This case illustrates that even a relatively minor amount of alcohol ingested less than two hours prior to going to bed can have profound consequences on breathing during sleep.

Many patients at St. Michael's have found that omitting an alcoholic beverage at dinnertime or later in the evening has eliminated their snoring.

How Does Alcohol Cause Snoring?

Over the past fifteen years, many researchers in sleep disorders medicine have studied the effect of alcohol on breathing during sleep. We now believe that alcohol worsens your breathing in two ways. First, it relaxes your throat muscles, narrowing your throat and making it collapse during sleep. This relaxation of the throat muscles has been demonstrated by Drs. Faiq Issa and Colin Sullivan of Australia and subsequently confirmed by many other investigators.

Alcohol also acts on the central nervous system to suppress the respiratory centers and the awakening mechanisms. It also dilates the blood vessels and thus increases swelling of the throat tissue.

You don't need to get drunk for the effects to occur; just a few drinks can do it. In fact, many times hangovers are not attributable totally to the alcohol but to disturbed sleep and waking up many times from unknown episodes of apnea.

Alcohol and Apnea

The biggest danger from alcohol is for people who have sleep apnea. Alcohol is known to trigger or aggravate episodes of sleep apnea, sometimes with violent snoring and snorting, sometimes with cessation of

---

DON'T USE ALCOHOL TO GET TO SLEEP

People who use alcohol in an attempt to help them sleep better are misguided. In nearly everyone, drinking alcohol late in the evening produces troubled sleep. The person usually wakes up many times throughout the night. In fact, in chronic alcoholics, sleep patterns are very abnormal, often with hundreds of awakenings per night.

And of course, there is not only the risk of poor quality sleep and snoring, but the danger of slipping into alcohol dependence. Many alcoholics say they started drinking regularly when they used alcohol to try to get to sleep at night.

---

breathing so severe as to cause heart arrhythmia. Serious sleep apnea can be life-threatening, especially if a person has a history of lung or heart disease.

A study at the University of Florida in Gainesville showed the relation between alcohol and apnea. Twenty men were given four shots of vodka within an hour before bedtime, and had their sleep monitored. They had five times more episodes of sleep apnea after drinking the alcohol than when they had not consumed alcohol. "For those already suffering from cardiac and pulmonary disease, even moderate drinking before bedtime presents a risk," the Florida researchers concluded.

For people who have either obstructive sleep apnea or central apnea, even a small amount of alcohol at night is inadvisable. If you have apnea and you want to drink, then drink earlier in the day.

Another study by Dr. Colin Sullivan in Australia had patients with apnea or snoring drink moderate amounts of wine or beer between 6 and 9 P.M. in amounts they considered normal for a social occasion. All of the patients showed substantially increased breathing abnormalities during sleep after drinking the alcohol, especially in the first two hours of sleep. Those who normally experienced only snoring with a small amount of alcohol clearly showed symptoms of apnea. Dr. Sullivan was particularly concerned about the dangerously low levels of oxygen in the blood on nights after alcohol consumption—levels so low one researcher said that if the levels dropped repeatedly during the night, it could cause permanent brain damage.

And one director of a sleep lab has said: "All these effects of heavy snoring make me wonder by how long John Wesley Hardin really shortened the life of that hotel guest."

Other Serious Sleeptime Dangers

In addition to relaxing the muscles of the throat and thus causing more snoring and more apnea, drinking alcohol at night results in a general shortage of oxygen in the body. The heart muscle, faced with this shortage of oxygen, may start contracting irregularly, and beating with an abnormal rhythm. In people who already have heart problems, this additional stress on the heart may lead to a serious arrhythmia, even death.

Another effect of alcohol is that it suppresses arousal responses during sleep. This means that you do not wake up quickly when there is a dangerous situation, such as severe shortage of oxygen. (This shortage is called *hypoxia*.) Not waking up prolongs the duration of hypoxic episodes, further endangering your life. This is particularly important if you already have a heart or lung disease such as chronic bronchitis or emphysema that causes shortage of oxygen at night.

And there's more. Many studies have shown that patients with sleep apnea are at increased risk for sleep-related motor vehicle accidents and near accidents. Other studies show that having two or more drinks per day puts drivers at an increased risk of accidents and near accidents. What happens if you put them together? Drs. Michael Aldrich and Ronald Chervin, of the University of Michigan, found that persons studied who had apnea and took two or more drinks per day were *five times more* at risk of sleep-related accidents.

What to Do

The bottom line: if you snore or have insomnia or episodes of stopped breathing, don't drink and sleep.

Becoming a nondrinker is easy for some, difficult for others. There are good reasons it's not easy. For many years, our culture has made

---

FATAL COCKTAILS

Other substances that cause relaxation of the throat muscles are sleeping pills and muscle relaxants. These substances should *never* be combined with alcohol at night. Never! It can lead to serious side effects and can even be fatal.

drinking alcohol the thing to do. The peer pressure is especially strong for teenagers. It's considered cute or manly to drink too much and brag about it later. Even as we mature, our culture still often equates drinking with sociability, relaxation, and fun. Often that's where the good times are.

However, times are changing. More and more people are choosing not to drink, or to drink only one or two glasses of wine or beer with a meal. They've read the statistics of how drinking alcohol increases their risk of breast cancer, heart disease, liver failure, pancreatitis, dilated blood vessels of the esophagus, stomach ulcers, hemorrhage of the gastrointestinal tract, and dementia. And they find when they don't drink alcohol, they feel better the next day.

If you're a snorer, you can choose not to drink at all, or to drink only moderately and occasionally, but it's important not to drink heavily or within a couple of hours of going to sleep.

The Plan

As with smoking, you can go off alcohol at once, cold turkey, or you can eliminate it gradually from your life. If you usually have several drinks a night, you may find it difficult to stop all at once, and you may want to withdraw gradually. Cut down to one drink per night for a few nights, then to one very weak drink for a few nights. Then eliminate the alcohol completely and have a glass of fruit juice with ice instead.

You may find it easiest to eliminate or cut down on alcohol at the same time you eliminate cigarettes, because consuming one often triggers the desire for the other. In fact, we've recently learned that consuming alcohol not only increases psychological craving, it actually increases the *physical* craving to smoke. It works as a psychological cue to light up automatically from habit and also increases craving by its pharmacological action.

As with becoming a nonsmoker, extra attention to nutrition and exercise helps. Take a vitamin-mineral supplement that has plenty of calcium, magnesium, folic acid, vitamin B_6, and glutamine, and eat protein snacks frequently to help stabilize energy levels.

The Reward

When a heavy alcohol user stops drinking, often sleep can improve and snoring can stop in as little as two weeks; although depending on the length of time that you've been using alcohol, it may take longer. As they withdraw, some chronic alcohol users may have more insomnia than usual, and more frequent awakenings and sometimes nightmares. Often heavy users will resume drinking simply to protect themselves against these withdrawal symptoms. Be careful that you don't fall into that trap—give yourself plenty of time, and get professional help if you think you need it. Help is available at most health departments, hospitals, and mental health clinics. Or go to a meeting of Alcoholics Anonymous and check out its program. It's free.

Motivate yourself by remembering that heavy drinkers have an overwhelmingly higher incidence of high blood pressure, stomach and duodenal ulcers, asthma, diabetes, gout, stroke, pancreatic disease, and certain cancers. Alcohol often causes headaches, diarrhea, insomnia, and irritability. It decreases sexual performance, and it robs you of feeling good the next day.

Keep your cocktail hour if it's important to you, but instead of alcohol have snacks, nonalcoholic beverages, and great music and conversation. Instead of a nightcap before going to bed, have a fruit juice or bedtime tea, such as chamomile. One couple talked to friends with whom they met frequently and asked them whether they would be interested in drinking less at their get-togethers, and were surprised to find that the others said it would be a relief to get out of the drinking rut.

And remember, not being drunk doesn't mean you have to be a wallflower. Live it up! Get a natural high from your own good spirits and the camaraderie of those around you.

If a party's so dull you need to have another drink to stand it, leave the party. Or see if that person in the corner also looking bored would like to take a walk and find something more fun to do.

As you did when you stopped smoking, and as you should do in any change program, reward yourself. Take the money you've saved and go buy something you've wanted or do something special. At the very least you will reward yourself—and your bedpartner—with more restful sleep.

5

Nutrition and Exercise

A 28-year-old woman—we'll call her Sue—came to St. Michael's Hospital because of her snoring. Sue had been married for three years. Her husband said that before they were married and for the first half of their marriage she snored, but not much, and he had not considered it a problem. But during the last eighteen months she had gained more than 50 pounds and her snoring had become very bad. To allow him to rest, she would go to sleep in a different room, wait until her husband fell asleep, and then join him in bed. But at least four nights a week, he would wake up in the middle of the night because of her loud snoring and he would leave the bedroom. In the morning he was usually irritable and fatigued. After four years of musical beds, the marriage ended.

Sam's story had a happier ending. He was a 48-year-old very obese man, weighing 396 pounds, who had been a heavy snorer for many years. Sam's snoring was so bad that most nights his wife slept in another room. In fact, Sam's snoring was so loud that even his dog, a German shepherd very devoted to him, could not sleep in the same room. Sam's snoring was so loud that when he stayed in a hotel in Connecticut on a business trip, so many guests complained of his snoring (even those not in adjoining rooms) that the hotel manager asked him not to come back. Sam tried a system called nasal CPAP, which eliminated his snoring, but he was unwilling to use it on a regular basis. (CPAP is explained in a later chapter.) He also tried a dental appliance, which reduced his snoring, but he found it uncomfortable. He was not a good candidate for surgery because of other physical conditions. After several visits to the clinic, he decided to participate in a weight-reduction program. In eight months on a weight-reduction diet, he lost 88 pounds and his snoring was greatly reduced. A sleep study showed that instead of 980 snores per hour of sleep he now had only 230 snores per

61

hour; furthermore, his snoring was no longer continuous throughout the night, but only sporadic. His wife and his dog both moved back into the bedroom.

Sam's case illustrates two points. First, weight loss reduces snoring. Second, you may not have to get your weight all the way down to your ideal body weight to see an improvement in snoring. Sam is still obese, but less so than he was before. He had lost enough weight to make a difference in his snoring.

Weigh Less, Snore Less

Being overweight is the most common cause of snoring. And if you are overweight and snore, getting down to a normal weight is often the only thing you need to do to eliminate your snoring.

Although the sleep disorders center at St. Michael's Hospital has a multidisciplinary approach to snoring, experience over the years has shown that the one thing that makes the biggest difference in helping overweight patients to stop snoring is to lose weight. It is also the most important thing to do to treat episodes of apnea.

If you snore a *little* and you gain weight, chances are that your snoring will progressively worsen—especially if you also smoke cigarettes, or if you use alcohol or sleeping pills at night. And if you continue to be overweight, you will begin to get symptoms of apnea. If you continue to gain weight, your apnea will get more and more severe. It is only a question of time.

How Excess Weight Can Cause Snoring or Make It Worse

When you are overweight, you usually have a fat neck. Increased neck circumference is one of the strongest correlates of snoring and apnea. If your shirt size is greater than 17 and you snore, you should seriously consider finding out whether you have sleep apnea.

Being overweight causes snoring and apnea by altering the anatomy and functioning of the throat. The excess fat causes narrowing of the airways. Since the fat is usually deposited along the sides of the throat or all around it, it can cause concentric narrowing of the throat, or it may simply encroach on the upper airway space. There have been numerous studies in which patients with sleep apnea had CAT scans or MRI images of their throats, all of which demonstrated that people with apnea had greater fat deposits than people without apnea.

Probably an even more important reason why being overweight leads to snoring and apnea is that increased fat within the muscles of the throat causes increased floppiness and collapsibility of the tissues of the throat. As you breathe in, the floppy walls move inward, narrowing the throat, and begin to vibrate, causing snoring. In addition, the presence of fat may impair the connections between the muscles of the throat and the rest of the tissues, so that when muscles contract, trying to stiffen the walls of the throat, the tissues in the walls respond poorly, resulting in continuing floppiness of the tissues.

Weight loss definitely improves snoring and apnea, as many studies have shown, but the exact mechanism is still only speculation. We know that snoring and apnea are a result of a narrow throat and floppy tissues in the airway, so losing weight is thought to improve those conditions and strengthen the walls of the throat. If you are obese, you have a thick neck, with lots of fatty tissue under the chin. When you lie down and go to sleep and the muscles of the throat relax, it is possible that the weight of this extra fat further narrows the airway passage, making it more susceptible to collapse. Also, if you are obese, your lungs become smaller when you lie down because the weight of your belly pushes on your diaphragm, forcing it into the chest. This adds to the reduction of the airway in the throat.

At the University of Toronto, we studied twelve overweight patients with snoring and apnea who had surgery to reduce weight by removing part of the stomach (called *gastroplasty*). The area of the airway and the collapsibility of the throat tissues were measured before and after surgery. There was a highly significant decrease in floppiness: after surgery the walls of the throat were much stiffer and much less susceptible to collapse. This resulted in a marked reduction in snoring and stopped-breathing episodes, from 57 per hour of sleep before surgery to 14 per hour after surgery.

In general, if you reduce the circumference of the neck and improve the stability of your throat tissues by losing weight, snoring occurs less often, or may even disappear completely.

If you're overweight and you snore, you first should lose your excess weight with a sound program of diet and exercise, and see what the results are from that before you take any serious medical or surgical action against snoring. Or if you and your doctor decide you need to have surgery or use CPAP, you should also work together on a weight-loss and fitness program to make that treatment more effective.

But how do you know if losing weight will help *you*? If you were not always overweight, think back to when you weighed less. Your sleep apnea will probably disappear with weight loss if you did not snore or have symptoms of sleep apnea before you put on that weight.

How much weight should you lose? This depends in part on how bad your snoring or apnea are and how overweight you are. If you have snoring without apnea and are not very overweight, sometimes losing 10 pounds will make all the difference in the world. If you have mild apnea and are only about 20 pounds overweight, losing those 20 pounds can eliminate the apnea. But if you weigh, say, 300 pounds and have severe apnea, you may need to lose a lot to get your weight low enough to eliminate sleep apnea. The good news is that *whatever* weight you lose, it will help; and the closer you get to your normal weight, the better your chance of eliminating your snoring.

Weight loss is the most natural form of treatment for snoring and apnea. It doesn't require any medicines or devices or surgery. And as a bonus, losing weight is also good for your heart and vascular system, decreases your chances of a heart attack, and helps you have more energy and feel better.

The Evidence

Many studies have shown the relationship of excess weight to snoring. You will remember from the Tucson study mentioned earlier that cigarette smoking, nighttime use of alcohol and sleeping pills, and obesity were all found to be factors in snoring. The specific statistics were that the prevalence of snoring in obese subjects was *three times* higher than in others, for both men and women. In several studies conducted by Dr. Poul Jennum and colleagues in Copenhagen, Denmark, hundreds of people were interviewed and asked questions about their snoring, diet, physical activity, alcohol consumption, and other factors. It was found and reported in 1995 that as a group, snorers weighed more than nonsnorers, exercised less, and consumed more alcohol. Similar results were found by Dr. Markku Koskenvuo and colleagues in Finland, who surveyed 3,750 men and found that a man who was 5 feet 9 inches tall and weighed 192 pounds was almost twice as likely to snore as a man who weighed less than 192 pounds.

Being overweight is a big factor in apnea also. Drs. Christian Guilleminault and William Dement as early as 1978 found that approximately two-thirds of patients with sleep apnea were obese, that is, at least 130 percent of their ideal body weight. An even more striking result was found by Dr. Terry Young and coworkers in Madison, Wisconsin. In one of the most widely quoted epidemiological studies regarding the prevalence of sleep apnea in the general population, these researchers found that if you are 5 feet 8 inches tall, do not have sleep apnea, and do not snore, but you gain weight, then for each 37 pounds of weight gain, you increase your risk of sleep apnea by more than four times.

According to the National Center on Sleep Disorders Research, approximately three out of every four cases of obstructive sleep apnea are caused by obesity. Data from a Cleveland study suggest that obese subjects are more than three times more likely to have apnea than are nonobese people.

The examples of obese patients whose apnea and snoring resolves or significantly improves after weight loss are numerous. In 1995 Drs. Howard Braver, A. Jay Block, and Michael Perri, of Gainesville, Florida, studied snoring treated with weight loss, sleeping on the side, and nasal sprays. The greatest improvement came with weight loss. All patients who lost *any* weight reduced their snoring to some degree, and the patients who lost 7.6 kg (171 pounds) or more virtually eliminated snoring completely. Dr. Anne Decary and others from the University of Montreal in Canada describe a 34-year-old patient who weighed 281 pounds and had severe snoring and apnea. He had partial restriction of his stomach by surgery and subsequently lost 120 pounds. His apnea episodes disappeared completely. He also saw significant improvement in attention, memory, and mental functioning.

About three out of every four people with sleep apnea are overweight, according to Dr. Paul Suratt, director of the Sleep Center at the University of Virginia Medical Center and a founder of the American Sleep Apnea Association. He says that in overweight patients, weight loss will almost always improve their apnea, and if enough weight is lost, sleep apnea will be completely eliminated in most people. He and other researchers at the University of Virginia found in one study of eight people with apnea that six saw significant improvement in apnea and all experienced less daytime sleepiness after losing weight.

How Overweight Are You?

There are several ways to judge whether you are overweight. One is to take off your clothes and look in the mirror. Another is to do the pinch test: Pinch a piece of skin between your fingers near your waist. If you have more than "an inch of pinch," you are probably overweight.

Or use the rule of thumb: If you're a woman with a medium frame, calculate your ideal weight by figuring 100 pounds for the first 5 feet of your height, plus 5 pounds for every inch above 5 feet. A man with a medium frame should calculate his ideal weight by figuring 106 pounds for his first 5 feet, plus 6 pounds for every inch above that. People with small frames should subtract 10 percent from the total; those with large frames should add 10 percent. Tables of ideal weight can also be used to determine the best weight for a person of your height and build.

Body Mass Index

You can use tables of ideal weight to determine whether you are overweight, but most scientists don't talk of pounds or kilograms so much as they do body mass index (BMI), which is your weight divided by your height squared.

Here's how you can calculate your BMI yourself: If you live in a country that uses the metric system, first measure your height in meters and multiply that number by itself to get your height squared. Then get on a scale, record your weight in kilograms, and divide your weight by your height squared. This is your BMI. For example, if you are 1.7 m tall and weigh 70 kg, multiply 1.7 by 1.7 to get 2.89, then divide 70 by 2.89, giving a BMI of 24.2.

If you live in a country that uses the system of inches and pounds, you need to convert. Measure your height in inches and multiply it by itself. Then measure your weight in pounds and multiply it by a factor of 705. Divide this by your height squared to get your BMI. For example, suppose you are 5 feet 10 inches tall and weigh 170 pounds. Your height in inches is 70. Multiply 70 by itself to get 4,900. Take your weight, 170, and multiply by 705. Divide that number by 4,900, which gives you 24.5, your BMI.

Or you can use a chart, called a Normogram, shown on page 68. Find your height in column A. Find your weight in column B. Draw a line through the two spots and extend the line to column C. The number where the line meets column C is your BMI.

If your BMI is more than 25 but less than 27, it means you are "overweight."* If your BMI is greater than 27, you are obese. Some doctors reserve the term "obese" for those with a BMI greater than 30. "Morbidly obese" usually means a BMI greater than 40. A healthy range is between 20 and 25. It is important to note that BMI is designed for adults aged 20–65. It does not apply to babies, children, adolescents, pregnant or nursing women, senior citizens, very muscular people, or endurance athletes such as runners.

The Easiest Way

Another way to judge whether you are overweight is to use a body fat monitor. Instead of weighing yourself as with a scale, you enter in your height, gender, and age, and the body fat monitor sends an electrical signal through your body (called *bioelectrical impedance analysis*) and tells you your body fat percentage. For example, for a man over 30 years old, a healthy body fat range is 17 to 23 percent; for a woman over age 30, it is 20 to 27 percent.

But you do not have to keep track of your weight loss with any of these, or even a scale. Instead, as you eat differently and exercise more, notice how you look and feel better, how your belt fits more loosely, how you can fasten it one hole tighter, or how you can fit into some clothes banished to a corner of the closet because they got too tight.

A Diet and Exercise Program against Snoring

Our antisnoring diet and exercise program is designed for the person who snores and is overweight. If you use another method to lose weight and increase fitness, it will probably be satisfactory, but check with your physician. The guidelines to our diet and exercise plans are carefully

---

*The term "overweight" is properly used for persons who are up to 20 percent over their ideal weight. The term "obese" refers to being more than 20 percent over ideal weight. "Morbidly obese" means being more than 75 percent over ideal weight.

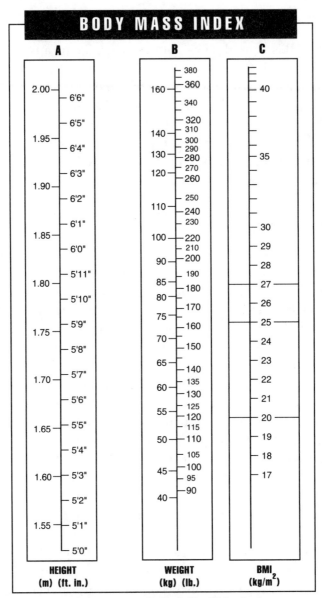

BODY MASS INDEX

A	B	C
HEIGHT (m) (ft. in.)	WEIGHT (kg) (lb.)	BMI (kg/m^2)

Adapted from a chart produced by Health and Welfare Canada.

formulated not only to help you lose weight in a way that works, but also to supply the nutrition and exercise that your body needs for good performance, and above all to be safe.

The program combines healthy eating and healthy exercise so that you are eliminating weight both by what you eat and by how well you metabolize it, and at the same time are using the nutrition and exercise to improve your cardiovascular system and your general health. We have also taken into consideration such things as keeping salt low to help eliminate tissue swelling, and avoiding foods that most frequently cause allergic reactions. The exercise part of the program not only is good for burning calories and speeding up metabolism, but also has beneficial antisnoring effects such as clearing up nasal congestion. In addition, weight loss and exercise will improve both your overall physical fitness level and your mental outlook.

And remember that when it comes to weight loss and nutrition, one size does not fit all. When you make your dietary decisions, keep in mind—and discuss with your doctor—any special medical conditions that you have as well as your family's medical history. For example, persons with a family history of cancer are usually advised to eat a lot of fruits and vegetables, as well as less fat and more fiber. Persons with a family history of heart disease, diabetes, or gallbladder disease are usually advised to cut down on sugar and eat a low-fat, high-fiber diet, with lots of whole grains, fruits and vegetables, and lean meat, fish, or poultry. Needs for calcium differ with age. The National Academy of Sciences has recently revised its recommendations to the following:

1 to 3 years: 500 mg per day

4 to 8 years: 800 mg per day

9 to 18 years: 1,300 mg per day

19 to 50 years: 1,000 mg per day

51 and older: 1,200 mg per day

Pregnant or lactating women should get 1,000–1,300 mg per day.

The best calcium sources are milk and milk products, broccoli, spinach, tofu, almonds, mustard greens, navy beans, turnips, and fortified foods such as orange juice. Calcium supplements should be quick-dissolving to be well-absorbed. The newly released report from the

National Academy of Sciences concludes that those at particular risk of developing osteoporosis should consume between 1,000 and 1,300 mg of calcium per day. Some others believe that women after menopause should take 1,400 to 2,000 mg of calcium per day. Calcium is best taken on an empty stomach.

You also need to work with your doctor if you try any special diets, such as those using a vegetable and fruit juice program or body-cleansing herbal supplements. If you use any diets that don't allow you to have a full array of food groups, then be sure to take recommended vitamin-mineral supplements so that you get adequate nutrients and keep your body in proper mineral balance.

Studies of people who have lost weight and kept it off show that some do it by restricting calories, others by cutting down on fat, others by cutting down on sugar and refined starches. We describe a diet that is healthy and that has been successful not just for losing weight, but in keeping it off long term. It is important for you to lose weight if you are overweight, but you also want to be eating for maximum health and energy, and to be able to enjoy eating.

The Ten-Step Weight-Loss Diet

The definition of "diet" is what you eat, but just as important is when and how you eat. Therefore, we give you not just recommendations for the kinds of foods to eat or not to eat to lose weight and reduce snoring, but also advice on how to eat them and when.

If you are overweight and you put into practice as much as possible our ten-step weight-loss diet, you should not only lose weight, but also as a result have a significant decrease in your snoring.

1. *Eat your largest meal at breakfast or lunch, your smallest meal at night.* Calories taken in earlier in the day are burned up faster because of your increased activity during the day, and fewer calories are stored as fat. If you have insomnia or snoring problems, you especially don't want a heavy meal sitting in your digestive system when you go to bed. It can bring on heavier sleep that will aggravate snoring, and a distended stomach can interfere with movement of the diaphragm, reducing breathing movement and worsening apnea.

   Healthy choices: Eat a large lunch, then have the leftovers or a large salad for dinner. If you work, take time for a large meal at lunch, which will also give you a stress break, then have something light and easy to fix for dinner, which will give you more time for friends and family. Be sure to include some protein in your dinner to help prevent hunger pangs in the night.

2. *Don't skip meals—instead eat mini-meals or snacks three, four, even five times a day or more.* You can eat as often as you want; just make the meals light and nutritious. People who skip meals often are so hungry that they eat more in the long run at the next meal. But more than that, studies have shown that apparently the same number of calories spread out over several meals are metabolized differently. One study showed that people eating 2,000 calories in a single meal gained weight, but when eating 2,000 calories spread over three or four meals, the same people *lost* weight.

Healthy choices: Stay away from junk food snacks, and instead grab some yogurt or shredded wheat cereal. Prepare snacks in the morning to graze on through the day: Put carrots and celery sticks in a bowl of water kept in the front of the refrigerator so it's easy to reach. Or keep cheese and crackers, apples, and raisins handy on the counter. You can graze all day without the hunger pangs that make you want to overeat. You can also prepare dinner in the morning: Make a big bowl of cole slaw using cabbage, carrots, and raisins, but only a tiny bit of mayonnaise, and garnish with slices of hard-boiled egg. Refrigerate till dinnertime.

3. *Eat as many vegetables and salads as possible, and as fresh as possible.* You can eat all you want of vegetables and salads. Buy them fresh, store them for as short a time as possible, and eat them raw or cook them in the least amount of water possible. Don't overcook them and don't let them sit after cooking.

Healthy choices: Asparagus, beans, broccoli, cabbage, cauliflower, cucumbers, greens, lettuce, spinach, squash, zucchini, carrots, celery, onions, peppers, tomatoes, and any other vegetable that you are not allergic to. Gorge on vegetables to your heart's content, four or five servings a day. (If you are a vegetarian, be sure to get adequate protein in your diet.)

4. *Eat lots of whole grain foods.* Eating a diet rich in whole grains can reduce your risk of heart disease, diabetes, and even certain types of cancer, as well as reduce cholesterol and triglyceride levels and lower high blood pressure. Eliminate white bread and other foods made from white flour and other refined starches. Filling up with fiber is a great way to satisfy your hunger.

   Healthy choices: Get your carbohydrates from potatoes and whole grain breads and cereals. Choose brown rice instead of white rice. Eat whole grain pasta and whole wheat or multi-grain crackers instead of products made with white flour. Make sure "bleached flour" isn't on the label. (One reason manufacturers bleach flour is that insects won't bother bleached flour so you can store it for a long time. If even the bugs know it isn't any good, why should you eat it?)

5. *Limit your intake of highly refined or highly processed foods.* Food manufacturers seem to put more and more chemicals into our food and take more and more vitamins and minerals out. Foods are not all created equal, so don't waste your taste. Eating fresh foods keeps the vitamins in and the additives out.

   Healthy choices: If possible, buy direct from a farmer who you know uses the old-fashioned methods of organic gardening. But that's not easy, so check out health food stores and the natural foods section of grocery stores for foods that have not been precooked, packaged with chemical preservatives, dyes, and artificial colors, or otherwise processed.

6. *Limit your intake of salt and other sodium.* Cutting out salt was once thought to be important in lowering high blood pressure, but research now indicates that being a normal weight, eating lots of fruits and vegetables, and exercising are more important in lowering blood pressure. However, there is another reason for limiting salt and other sodium: Less salt intake helps prevent fluid buildup that often causes overweight people to have edema. And less tissue swelling in the airway passages can mean less snoring.

   Healthy choices: Read the labels. Limit your intake of the many foods and beverages that have sodium in them. Don't add a lot of salt to your food.

7. *Eliminate sugar as much as possible.* The average person eats more than 100 pounds of sugar per year. Sugar is high in calories, has no food value, and has been implicated in many health problems. Read labels and stay away from products with sugar. Sugar can be sucrose, dextrose, glucose, lactose, maltose, or corn syrup. Don't use sugarcoated cereals or sugared soft drinks.

Healthy choices: Get whatever sugar you want from the natural sugars in fresh fruits. Choose unsweetened juices. If you use canned or frozen fruits, buy the ones that are packed in water or natural juices, not syrup. Break the habit of automatically having a sweet dessert after a meal and instead have your salad at the end of the meal. Have something sweet only occasionally as something special that you really want.

8. *Limit your intake of fat.* Many people crave fat as much as they crave sugar. But it has been shown that a low-fat diet can not only help you lose weight, it can also lower your risk of heart disease and certain cancers. Watch for hidden fat in cakes, cookies, doughnuts, ice cream, and candies. Notice that we did not say to give up fat completely. You need a certain amount to produce your body hormones and to help you feel full.

Healthy choices: Trim the fat off poultry and meat, eat more fish and poultry instead of meat, avoid gravies and rich sauces, order foods that are baked or broiled instead of fried, and only use a small amount of salad dressing. Plan some meals around beans and rice instead of meat. Choose skim or 2 percent milk instead of whole milk. You don't have to give up eggs if you have normal cholesterol levels; they are very nutritious.

9. *Limit your intake of alcohol, and never drink just before bed.* Alcohol has a lot of calories, and it can lead to hangovers, liver damage, and addiction. And important for the person who snores, it depresses the central nervous system and causes louder, heavier snoring. If you have apnea, it increases the severity of the stopped-breathing episodes.

Healthy choices: Have club soda with a lemon wedge, bottled water, or other nonalcoholic drink. To lessen calories, especially stay away from beer and sweet dessert wines and after-dinner liqueurs. And if you snore or have apnea remember to never, never, never drink alcohol just before you go to sleep.

10. *Drink a lot of water every day.* Water is incredible for helping you lose weight and, surprisingly, for decreasing fluid retention. It helps fill you up, but it does more than that. It helps your body metabolize fat faster and get rid of it. It helps the cells function better, helps rid the body of toxic wastes, and most important, it helps your body release and get rid of the stored water that causes fluid retention. Diet doctors report that patients who drink a lot of water lose weight faster than those who don't. Often when dieters are having trouble losing weight, increasing water intake is what finally makes the weight start to come off.

Healthy choices: Drink six or eight glasses of water or more per day. However, if you are not drinking this much water at present, you need to build up to that level gradually, increasing your intake by about one glass every other day. Drink the water even if you're not thirsty. Some people drink so little water that they lose their sense of thirst. It will come back.

Tips for Making Weight Loss Easier and Faster

Eat as varied a diet as possible. If you eat a variety of foods, it will keep you from getting bored and you will more likely be provided with the greatest variety of nutrients. No single food includes all nutrients, and we still don't know all the nutritional requirements of the body, so eating a varied diet will help increase your odds of getting what you need.

Here are some other quick tips:

- Find a friend and go on the ten-step weight-loss program together.
- Start a meal with a glass of water or a low-calorie soup.
- Drink water with your meal instead of a beverage that contains sugar.
- Watch not only what you cook, but also how you cook it.
- Serve food directly onto plates instead of putting the serving bowls on the table. This cuts down on second servings.
- Keep fattening food out of sight. Give away your candy dish and cookie jar, or at least put them out of sight to discourage walk-by snacking.

- In a buffet or cafeteria, check out the food choices before you select. You can make your choices more carefully.

- When you travel, take along low-calorie fruit, vegetable, or protein snacks.

- When you're hungry, take a walk. It will inhibit the hunger urge as well as burn up some calories.

- If you think it will be helpful, keep a food diary and mark down when you eat, including unplanned snacks, and the situations and feelings that preceded or accompanied any overeating binges.

- If you make a poor choice, don't feel guilty. Give yourself credit for all the good choices you've been making, and just get back

---

VITAMIN-MINERAL SUPPLEMENTS

It's best to get your nutrients in natural form, so follow a healthy diet that includes the greatest variety of the freshest foods possible. It is also a good idea to take vitamin-mineral supplements to ensure against nutritional deficiencies, especially if you are on a weight-loss diet. The diet of the average American adult tends to be especially deficient in iron, zinc, folic acid, and calcium. And many older persons also need extra vitamin D and B vitamins. If you are under stress because of not sleeping well, or because you are having difficulty eliminating cigarettes, alcohol, or sleeping pills from your life, then you may also want to try a vitamin B complex to help you deal with the stress. And since nearly everyone needs more calcium, taking a calcium supplement at bedtime not only helps strengthen bones and prevent osteoporosis, but also is a substitute for the sleeping pill habit.

If you have any special health problems, talk to your doctor and to a health food store consultant about some vitamin-mineral supplements that might be helpful. For example, if you have a high cholesterol level, you may be helped by taking vitamins A, B_3, B_6, and C, as well as pectin, lecithin, choline, inositol, calcium, magnesium, pangamic acid, manganese, and para-aminobenzoic acid (PABA). There are also specific vitamins and minerals for you to consider taking if you have insomnia.

in the groove of healthy choices. Remember, the goal is reached over the long run, and it's one meal at a time, one snack at a time, one holiday dinner at a time that will eventually make the difference.

- Continue to enjoy eating; just eat the right things. As you gain control over your eating and your life, you will feel new self-confidence and new energy, and best of all, as the pounds drop, you will find that you snore less.

If You Think You Have a Food Allergy

More and more, food allergies are being diagnosed, according to a recent report of the AMA, but researchers are not sure whether the increase is actual or due to greater awareness and reporting of allergies. Currently, it is estimated that food allergies affect about 1.5 percent of the adult U.S. population (and 6 percent of infants).

Many allergic reactions are avoided on our recommended diet because you will eat mostly fresh, unprocessed foods.

Food allergies, like other allergies, can cause nasal congestion or fluid retention in the body, and you know both of those things are not good for you if you snore, so be on the lookout for any foods that might do this to you.

Often the very things you crave are the things that you are allergic to. Keep track. You may get withdrawal symptoms when you stop eating a food you are allergic to, much like you get when you go off caffeine or sugar, with headache, irritability, or tension. Many times people keep going back to the foods they are intolerant of just to get relief from the withdrawal symptoms.

If you think you are allergic to something, sometimes it helps to eat that food on a rotation plan: don't eat the same food that you are suspicious of more often than once every five days.

The foods most commonly associated with food allergy are milk, corn, wheat, chocolate, nuts, egg whites, seafood, and red and yellow food colorings. If you are allergic to any of these, be careful of their relatives, too. For example, if you are allergic to corn, you may also be allergic to corn starch, corn syrup, sorbitol, mannitol, and dextrose, all of which are made from corn.

If you are allergic to meat, you may find it helpful to substitute soy

---

WHAT ABOUT CAFFEINE?

Ordinarily the person trying to lose weight is better off eliminating caffeine from the diet because of the relation between caffeine's metabolic effects and food cravings. And if you have insomnia, you need to stay away from caffeine. But snoring occurs most often during the cycles of deep sleep, so it can sometimes be beneficial to use caffeine to lighten sleep and keep out of the deeper cycles. Confusing? Our recommendation is that you experiment to see what works for you. Keep track of the caffeine you ingest in the form of coffee, soft drinks, and chocolate, and see how your snoring is affected with and without caffeine.

---

protein for animal protein. An added benefit is that it has been shown to help with weight loss, as well as lower cholesterol and triglycerides. Soy protein is found in soy milk and tofu.

By the way, skin tests are not reliable for diagnosing food allergies. They give many false positives to foods that you are not actually allergic to. You simply have to keep track of foods and see which ones you have a reaction to.

The Good News

If you are overweight, you are at higher risk of heart disease, stroke, diabetes, and high blood pressure. If you get your weight to normal, you will reduce all these risks. And you will look and feel better and have more energy. In addition, the AMA recently announced that avoiding weight gain can help prevent breast cancer.

The benefits of not being fat have been shown over and over by scientific studies. For example, a nationwide study by the National Heart, Lung, and Blood Institute, showed that when patients followed a diet low in saturated fats and rich in dairy products, fruits, and vegetables, their blood pressure was lowered. The study showed that if you have high blood pressure, as many people with snoring and apnea do, a diet consisting of eight to ten servings of fruits and vegetables a day with one or two servings of dairy products can lower your blood pressure as much as some drug therapy. "Once again we've learned that what your mother always told you was right," says Dr. George Bray, one of the principal investigators in the study.

What about Diet Pills?

First there were amphetamines such as Dexedrine that people used because they suppressed appetite, but they proved to be addictive. Then came the new weight-loss pills Pondimin (fenfluramine) and Redux (dexfenfluramine), most often paired with phentermine, another weight-loss medication, in a combination called "fen-phen." The pills were designed for people who were seriously overweight (at least 30 percent over their healthy body weight), not for people who wanted to just drop 10 pounds or so. But millions used the pills—doctors called the craze "fen-phen fever." In fact, some 18 million prescriptions were written in 1996 for fen-phen at the peak of the fad.

The pills were used in Europe for many years, and are still available in various combinations in many countries. But problems began to show up. The drugs were found to alter brain chemistry. If Redux was taken with monoamine oxidase (MOA) inhibitors, often used to treat depression or Parkinson's disease, it was found that the combination of drugs could cause serious, sometimes fatal reactions. Doctors from the National Institute of Mental Health in Bethesda, Maryland, warned in the *Journal of the American Medical Association (JAMA)* that physicians and patients also needed to be alert for such things as memory loss, irregular moods, anxiety, aggression, and changes in sleep patterns (although these symptoms may have many causes).

In 1994, an alert technician in Fargo, North Dakota, found leaky heart valves on echocardiograms of two women taking fen-phen. In late 1997, Mayo Clinic physicians found a form of heart valve disease in twenty-four women taking fen-phen. Five of the women needed heart surgery to repair the damaged valves. Eight were found to have pulmonary hypertension (a serious condition in which the blood pressure in the arteries supplying the lungs is abnormally high). Then physicians learned of sixty-one more cases, and possibly some deaths. The Food and Drug Administration (FDA) issued an advisory—a "Dear Doctor" letter—after their hotline received other reports of psychosis, seizures, depression, hallucinations, and amnesia in fen-phen users. Experts warned that the drug should not be used in patients with existing mental problems. Then another group of doctors found nearly one-third of 291 patients taking the drugs had unrealized heart valve irregularities. The FDA requested that the manufacturers pull the drug off the market, and they have voluntarily recalled the pills from drugstore shelves.

An article in the June 1997 issue of *JAMA* warns that many weight-loss products can cause side effects. For example, a fat substitute called Olestra can cause cramps or diarrhea. Others warn that Dexatrim and Acutrim should not be taken by anyone with high blood pressure. The herb ephedra (ma huang) contains ephedrine, which stimulates the nervous system and the heart, and is being investigated as a possible cause of upsets in heart rhythm, rapid pulse, increased blood pressure, dizziness, headache, and insomnia. And the FDA cautions that the new drug Meridia should not be taken by people with poorly controlled high blood pressure, heart disease, or irregular heartbeat, or by those who have had a stroke.

Two common ingredients in over-the-counter weight-loss formulas are chromium picolinate, which plays a role in insulin action and carbohydrate and fat metabolism, and *Garcinia cambogia,* made from a fruit that is native to India. Herbs sometimes used are *Polygonum multiflorum, Hypericum,* and *Alisma rhizoma.* At the time this book went to press, no bad side effects had been reported with any of these but they are being researched further for safety.

The truth is there are few long-term studies on the safety of diet pills. If you use any of them, or any new diet pills that come on the market, don't pop them like candy, don't take more than the recommended dosage, investigate to see whether there are any reported side effects, and only use them after consulting with your doctor.

And remember, diet pills are not magic cures to be used alone, but are to be used along with a diet and exercise program. It's best to lose weight without pills, but if you do use them remember that you still have to change your habits. And when you stop the pills, there's no guarantee the weight you lost will stay off unless you've made major lifestyle changes to eat the right foods and eat moderately, and stick to a calorie-burning exercise program.

The Role of Exercise

Poor physical fitness in addition to obesity has been found by some investigators to be related to snoring and apnea. Dr. Joseph Norman and others from the University of Nebraska Medical Center in Omaha were the first to study the usefulness of an exercise training program for managing symptoms of apnea. At the meeting of the Association of Professional Sleep Societies in 1997, they reported on six men who participated in an aerobic and strength-training exercise program three times a week for six months in addition to receiving dietary counseling for weight loss. The men lost an average of 17 pounds, their apnea symptoms disappeared or diminished, and they had better moods in their awake time.

The lack of exercise can creep up on you. You may have exercised actively in the past, but only a little decrease can make a difference. In the journal *Military Medicine* in 1997, Captain Larry Sonna, Dr. Philip Smith, and Dr. Alan Schwartz, of Baltimore, reported two cases of soldiers who snored so loudly that they were a threat to detection of their unit in field conditions. One snorer was a 52-year-old infantryman in the National Guard who put multiple layers of camouflage and netting on his encampment and slept at a site deep in the bush away from the rest of the soldiers in his unit because he didn't want to compromise their position. He was so sleepy during the day and while driving that his previous unit had called him "Sergeant Sleepy." His snoring was so loud and disturbed his wife so much that she wore earplugs and he began to work the night shift at his civilian job in a textile factory so his wife could sleep at night. He had been gaining weight progressively—a 40-pound weight gain in one year—which he attributed to insufficient exercise.

Sonna and his colleagues caution that there may be a significant number of cases of sleep apnea in the military and that medical personnel should suspect this condition in soldiers who have large body mass and are sleepy during the day or have unexplained poor performance. They suggest that snoring and sleep apnea could hinder performance of a military occupation and suggest tightening of army weight standards.

The Antisnoring Exercise Program

Lack of exercise is one of the chief reasons why most dieters fail in their weight-loss program, and exercise is the one thing that can help you lose weight most easily and quickly. In fact, not being a couch potato is probably more important than not eating french fries or potato chips. In a study of people who had gone on diets, lost weight, and kept it off, 90 percent had also modified their exercise habits, increasing their physical activity while they decreased their eating.

Remember that increased physical activity will help you burn more calories, will improve your adherence to the diet program, and will speed up your metabolism.

It's not just scheduled sports and training times themselves that burn more calories, improve your muscle tone, and increase your metabolic rate, but it's increased physical activity in general that can make a difference in your weight loss.

In fact, if you don't exercise, even if you eat less, you may not lose weight. Studies have shown that overweight people who are inactive and don't exercise actually have decreased basal metabolism rates—which means even if you eat less, your body burns the food more slowly and so puts on more weight.

One study showed that a group of overweight teenaged girls consumed fewer calories per day than thin teenaged girls. However, the overweight girls were far less active. They slept or sat almost five hours more per day than the thin girls. The difference was exercise.

Exercise enough and you can eat more and still be slimmer!

And don't worry about whether exercise will increase your appetite. The fact is that moderate exercise not only helps burn fat, but also helps inhibit the urge to eat. Believe it, with exercise, you will lose weight faster. This has been shown scientifically. In a study directed by Dr. George Blackburn of Harvard Medical School, it was shown that over a seven-week period among people eating 1,000 calories a day, those who exercised lost two and a half times as much weight as those who did not exercise. The next time you are at a party or a meeting, look around at the people. The overweight people hardly move, conserving energy. The thin ones move around much more.

The first thing you can do on your weight-loss program is to start putting more movement and activity into everyday life. Don't just sit there, do something to burn calories. Every movement burns some calories. Walk instead of riding. Take the stairs instead of the elevator. Walk more briskly when you are shopping. Rise up and down on your toes while waiting. Use a rocking chair while reading. Do stretching exercises during your coffee break and when taking a break at your desk. Park away from the entrance and walk. Swing your arms. Sway to the music. Something as simple as switching from a typewriter to a computer in a year's time can amount to a weight gain, and simply climbing the stairs every day instead of taking the elevator can make a similar difference in weight loss.

The second part of your exercise program is to start a regular pulse-raising (aerobic) exercise schedule and stick to it. Get involved in walking, bicycling, tennis, swimming, dancing, or some other activity you think is fun, and put it on a regular schedule so you will be motivated to stick with it. You will get the most benefit from aerobic exercise, not only because it burns calories, but also because it will increase your circulation, improve your heart and lung function, build stronger bones, tone muscles, reduce cholesterol levels, and increase the activity of your glands. People who exercise regularly have been shown to have less breast cancer, less arthritis, less high blood pressure, lower cholesterol, less osteoporosis, and better sleep. Studies by Dr. Abby King and colleagues of Stanford University School of Medicine in California found that thirty to forty minutes of brisk walking or low-impact aerobics four times per week cut in half the time needed to fall asleep, and patients claimed to be less tired in the morning.

People who have insomnia often are sedentary and don't exercise much. Regular exercise helps them go to sleep more easily and sleep better. People who always feel tired say with exercise they suddenly feel energized. With exercise you not only increase your general physical fitness and muscle tone, but also look and feel better. Exercising *will* help you lose weight, and losing weight *will* help cure snoring and apnea. Not bad for exercising an hour or two a week.

EXERCISE TIPS

Walking is one of the simplest, least expensive, and safest exercises. For weight loss, walk briskly, don't just stroll. The faster you walk, the more calories you will burn. Raining? Walk at the mall.

Time yourself. Start out gradually. Build up both your time and your distance. Be sure to start out slowly. If you start out doing too much too fast, it can result in muscle and joint pain and discourage you from continuing. Start gradually, and increase your activity slowly, step by step.

If your pulse becomes irregular or you feel dizzy or breathless, you should stop. Otherwise, keep progressively extending yourself to increase your metabolism even more, burn even more calories, and build stamina, fitness, and muscle tone.

6

Snoring and Medications

John was a 53-year-old executive working at a major financial institution. He had always had a problem with snoring, and his wife coped with it by sometimes wearing earplugs, sometimes poking him at night to make him turn on his side. Sometimes he would just decide to sleep in another room. For about three months prior to his visit to St. Michael's, John began to snore every night, louder than before, and his wife noticed, for the first time, episodes of apnea. She became alarmed and insisted that John seek medical attention. In taking his history, it soon became apparent that for the past several months John had been under a great deal of tension. His company was restructuring and John was worried about losing his job. He began having difficulties with sleep. Whereas before he would fall asleep as soon as his head hit the pillow, now he was lying awake for hours, worrying about his future. In the morning he felt tired and groggy, and his job performance was suffering, further compounding his worries. To sleep better and feel more rested in the morning, he started taking an occasional sleeping pill. Pretty soon it became a habit and he was taking them nightly. That was when his wife noticed his snoring worsened and his stopped-breathing episodes began. His sleep test showed that he snored loudly and frequently, and had twenty-three episodes of stopped or reduced breathing per hour of sleep. It was difficult to convince John of the possibility that sleeping pills were responsible for his increased snoring and occasional apnea. In fact, it was only after his job situation clarified (he was told that he would remain with the company) that he agreed to go off the sleeping pills. Within one week his snoring returned to the previous levels and his wife no longer observed periods of apnea. A sleep study confirmed that he snored less, and now had only six episodes of disturbed breathing per hour of sleep.

How Do Certain Medications Cause Snoring?

If you snore, you should not take sleeping pills, tranquilizers, or muscle relaxants. These medications usually cause muscles to relax, including your throat muscles, which can become floppy. This looseness of throat tissues is a very important cause of snoring. In fact, the muscle-relaxing side-effect actions of sleeping pills, tranquilizers, and muscle relaxants can be so significant that they can turn a nonsnorer into a snorer, a light snorer into a heavy snorer, and a heavy snorer into a snorer with apnea.

The Evidence

There are a number of studies showing the effect of sleeping pills and tranquilizers on snoring and apnea. For example, Dr. Hartmut Schneider and a team of researchers at Philipps University in Marburg, Germany, and Dr. Christian Guilleminault, of Stanford University School of Medicine in Stanford, California, studied the effect of two different benzodiazepine pills on breathing during sleep in a number of different subjects in the sleep lab. These are commonly used pills for insomnia and jet lag. The researchers found that on nights when subjects took either of the sleeping pills, there were increases in time spent snoring, especially with the pill flunitrazepam during non-REM stages (nondreaming stages 2, 3, and 4) of sleep.

And remember the study by Dr. John Bloom and his colleagues in

---

OTHER SIDE EFFECTS OF SLEEPING PILLS

There may be other side effects, too. Sleeping pills can also cause impaired performance the next day. They can leave you groggy and with a hangover, less able to perform with speed and accuracy. Tests of people adding numbers, playing video games, copying drawings, making decisions, or remembering words have all shown their performance was never better with a sleeping pill than without. Many times a person's performance is worse because of grogginess.

Tucson that we told you about in chapter 4. They surveyed more than 2,000 people in the Tucson area and found that the prevalence of snoring was 24 percent in those who used alcohol or sleeping pills at bedtime versus 15 percent in nonusers.

Tranquilizers, which are basically the same thing as sleeping pills but not as strong, can also be a problem if you are a snorer. Dr. Maurice Ohayon and colleagues from several institutions recently conducted a very extensive telephone interview survey of almost 5,000 people in Great Britain, both men and women, aged 15–100, and found that taking anxiety-reducing drugs put them two to four times at higher risk of having the breathing pauses of apnea during sleep.

Even if you never snored before or never had apnea, you may start if you take sleeping pills or tranquilizers. One 37-year-old woman came to the St. Michael's sleep clinic because of difficulty staying asleep. Both she and her husband reported that she did not snore and did not have stopped-breathing episodes, and nothing in her medical history suggested either snoring or apnea. She was not overweight, and she did not drink in the evenings, but she woke up a lot in the middle of the night and was tired in the daytime. She was sent to the sleep lab for an overnight study, and surprisingly her sleep study showed that she snored heavily and had on average twenty-two complete and partial pauses in breathing per hour of sleep. This was totally unexpected, and when we saw her during follow-up, we asked her whether there was anything unusual about the day of her sleep study. She said that she was very nervous about going to the lab, afraid she would not be able to fall asleep, and contrary to our instructions, decided to take a sleeping pill prior to her arrival at the lab. We scheduled another sleep study and told her this time to follow instructions and not take sleeping pills, tranquilizers, alcohol, or other sleep aids. Her repeat sleep study demonstrated no snoring and only three episodes of incomplete cessation of breathing per hour of sleep. The reason for her difficulty in sleeping turned out to be that she went to bed at widely varying times. Following a regular sleep schedule solved her problems. She decided to no longer use tranquilizers or sleeping pills.

Dr. Wallace Mendelson, of the Cleveland Clinic, reported a case of a man who had two to eighteen apnea episodes per hour on no-pill nights—not considered anything to worry about—but had one hundred apnea episodes per hour on nights when he took a sleeping pill.

These side effects can occur with over-the-counter medications as well as with prescription drugs, so don't feel that you can use over-the-counter pills as a substitute for prescription drugs.

At one time sleeping pills and tranquilizers were the most widely prescribed medicines in the world. Now research in sleep medicine is showing how detrimental these pills can be. The facts on their overuse are reaching physicians and the public, and things are beginning to change. Sleeping pills and tranquilizers aren't so widely used now, but they are still overprescribed and overused. For example, it is estimated that in the past year, Americans spent $100 million on over-the-counter sleep remedies alone, plus more than $2 *billion* on prescription remedies. We don't have statistics from other parts of the world. Despite the fact that sleep experts and even manufacturers themselves only recommend occasional use, many people still use them every night. And some hospitals and nursing homes give their patients sleeping pills on a routine basis whether they have trouble sleeping or not—and whether it makes their snoring and apnea worse or not.

Remember that all sleeping pills and tranquilizers work by slowing down the central nervous system. In fact, they can impact on breathing during sleep in many ways: they may decrease the brain's central respiratory drive, cause throat muscles to relax more, increase upper airway resistance, and decrease the arousal response, particularly in older subjects. All of those things will make snoring and apnea worse.

The Danger of Mixing Alcohol and Sleeping Pills

Larry, aged 62, was a snorer and drank alcohol heavily, usually in the evenings. He was a frequent visitor to the emergency room of the local hospital, usually because of alcohol-related complications. During one of his admissions, the nurses noticed episodes of cessation of breathing. This eventually led to a sleep study, in which he was found to have obstructive sleep apnea. He was advised to stop using alcohol and was prescribed a nasal CPAP, a device to assist in breathing. He kept drinking, however, and used the CPAP only occasionally. His wife was taking minor tranquilizers, prescribed by her physician, and Larry sometimes also took them, saying that they were "good for his nerves." One evening, having drunk his usual gin and tonic, he went to bed. His wife recalls that he tossed and turned for almost an hour, unable to sleep, then got up, took two of her pills, and went back to bed. Sometime in the middle of the night she awoke because of unusual quietness. Her husband was lying still and did not respond when she called him. She checked him and discovered that he was dead. The autopsy showed cirrhosis of the liver and an enlarged heart, but no heart attack. The chances are that a combination of alcohol and tranquilizers caused a particularly severe episode of apnea, with a very low oxygen level, leading to arrhythmia and death.

Taking a sleeping pill or tranquilizer and then drinking alcohol can be incredibly dangerous. Each adds to the effects of the other. In some cases, even one glass of wine or beer can be dangerous.

And the effect is worse if you have apnea—the combination can be fatal. Cases of sudden death at night, without an obvious cause, were studied by Dr. T. Seppala and colleagues of Helsinki, Finland. They found that many of these people were heavy habitual snorers, consumed alcohol, and were taking various medications. It is a definite possibility that some of these people may have had sleep apnea, and this might have been the cause of their sudden death.

Kicking the Habit

If you are frequently taking sleeping pills or tranquilizers, you should kick the habit, no matter how difficult it is.

If you have been regularly taking sleeping pills or tranquilizers for insomnia, talk to your doctor about getting off them and then taper off gradually. Tapering off is important because if you suddenly stop taking them, you will have several days of really bad insomnia, and sometimes other side effects.

This difficulty in sleeping when you go off sleeping pills is called "rebound phenomenon," and the higher the dosage you were taking, the longer you tend to have withdrawal symptoms. And the rebound insomnia usually is actually worse than the insomnia you had before you started taking the pills. Depending on the type of sleeping pill you were taking, you could also have a great deal of dreaming, even nightmares. Thank goodness it's only temporary.

Other side effects that can occur if you withdraw cold turkey are fatigue, weakness, depression, jitteriness, changes in taste and smell, cramps, nausea, and headache.

Any kind of sleeping pill can cause a rebound problem, so you may well have withdrawal symptoms. But you need to go ahead and get off them. The few nights of discomfort you may have will be worth the effort. Just do it gradually.

If you have insomnia, we recommend that you read *No More Sleepless Nights* (John Wiley & Sons, 1996) by Dr. Peter Hauri of the Mayo Clinic and Dr. Linde. This book contains many helps to treating insomnia and other sleep disorders without using pills.

How to Do It

Here are some tips on getting off sleeping pills by gradual withdrawal:

1. Give yourself extra help by learning relaxation techniques and other helpful nondrug techniques for fighting insomnia.

2. Pick a specific time to quit, giving yourself at least four weeks for withdrawal. Some people pick a vacation as a nonstress time. Others figure they might as well go through withdrawal during a stressful time and get it over with.

3. Announce your plan to others. Talk about the anticipated "last day of pill bondage." Announcing your plan to all who care will help you stick to it later.

4. Make a specific withdrawal plan. Keep only the medication that you have scheduled to use to get through your withdrawal period. Give the excess to a trusted friend to hold on to. To take a dose smaller than one pill, cut the tablet with a sharp knife into smaller and smaller pieces. If the pills come in capsule form, open the capsule, remove some of the contents, and put the capsule back together, then each week remove more until you get down to nothing. The first week, cut down by one-fourth the dosage that you now take. Each week after that, cut down to half of what you took the week before, until you are down to just a little dust for the last week. If you have difficulties with this plan, take smaller steps and stretch your withdrawal over six to eight weeks; but whatever step you have reached, don't allow yourself to go back to a higher dosage.

5. Have on hand a supply of books or materials for a favorite hobby to get you through the possible nights of sleeplessness. Continue your exercise, relaxation training, and social life.

Think about how much better your sleep is going to be and how much better you will feel in the daytime from now on.

6.   On the day of the last pill, have a celebration and flush away all the leftover pills.

You May Need Help

If withdrawal by yourself is too difficult, you may have to work with a doctor or other professional, or even spend a week or longer in a hospital where you can get medical and counseling support. Take the time to do it; it's important. In fact, it is so important that some sleep disorders centers have their own counseling services to help you become a nonuser, and many others are affiliated with other departments at their hospital or with nearby institutions specializing in drug addiction. A multispecialist team, usually headed by a psychiatrist or psychologist, will interview you, try to uncover the reason for your drug dependence, and initiate the treatment modality most appropriate for your individual situation.

Muscle Relaxants Can Be a Problem, Too

Like sleeping pills and tranquilizers, muscle relaxants (which you might take for back spasm or other muscle problems) can also cause the throat muscles to relax. So if you are a snorer, it may be helpful to eliminate not only sleeping pills and tranquilizers, but muscle relaxants as well. This is especially important if you are a heavy snorer or have apnea. Muscle relaxants can be as dangerous as sleeping pills and tranquilizers.

One 44-year-old woman came to St. Michael's sleep clinic because her heavy snoring was interfering with her marital life. Her snoring was so bad that for the past year her husband had not shared the same bedroom with her. Although she had snored for many years, it was only during the past year that her snoring had become very loud, frequent, and disruptive to her husband. She had sustained neck and back injuries in an automobile accident fourteen months earlier, and was in such constant pain that she was no longer able to work. She was undergoing physical therapy, and in addition was started on muscle relaxants, pain pills, and antidepressants. She had gained 35 pounds. When told that weight gain and the pills were contributing to her snoring, she said she needed the pills in order to function during the day. She was started on psychotherapy to help her overcome her dependence, and after two months she was able to discontinue the muscle relaxants. Within three weeks her husband noticed a marked reduction in her snoring, despite the fact that her weight remained the same and she still used pain pills and antidepressants. And he moved back into their bedroom.

Don't forget, by the way, that muscle relaxants can come in both prescription and over-the-counter forms. And both can cause problems.

Antihistamines and Other Medicines

Some antihistamines and other medicines, far too numerous to list here, can sometimes affect breathing and snoring. Sometimes the side effects occur regularly, sometimes in only some people.

The good news is that often new drugs or new forms of drugs come along that don't cause the side effects. For example, some tranquilizers and muscle relaxants have recently been shown not to worsen snoring. If you snore and are taking some kind of medicine, or if a new medicine is prescribed for you, discuss with your physician and your pharmacist what the possible side effects are and whether the medicine is likely to affect snoring or apnea. And always read the labels and accompanying literature with any medicines that you receive.

Do Any Medicines Help Snoring or Apnea?

It's logical to think that some type of medicine should be useful in relieving snoring and apnea. Since snoring and apnea occur in certain stages of sleep, why not a drug that alters sleep stages? And since apnea can be related to a reduced drive to breathe during sleep, why not a medicine to alter the drive to breathe?

A number of drugs using these approaches were tried, most of them for treatment of apnea rather than just for snoring.

For nasal obstruction, doctors tried nasal anti-inflammatory agents, decongestants, and antihistamines. Sometimes these work, but not always. It was found that intranasal steroids reduced inflammation in about 10 percent of snorers, particularly those with nasal stuffiness due to allergies. At the clinic at St. Michael's, we recommend intranasal steroids as a trial treatment for snoring patients who have nasal symptoms. We always warn patients, however, that they must exercise caution against prolonged use of these agents because it can lead to worsening of symptoms.

Snoring and apnea are more common in people with certain hormone abnormalities. For example, people with hypothyroidism (low thyroid) have a reduced drive to breathe and frequently develop apnea. In addition they usually have a large and bulky tongue, which may block the airway. Treatment with thyroid hormone will reverse the hormone abnormality and resolve snoring and apnea. However, snorers without thyroid disorder should not take this medication to get rid of snoring; it will not work, and could be dangerous.

Another hormone abnormality sometimes associated with apnea and snoring is acromegaly, a hormone disorder characterized by enlargement of all tissues. People with this disorder are usually tall and have large hands, bones, and facial structures, including a large tongue that can occlude the airway. Treatment of acromegaly is by medication or surgery or both, and snoring and apnea usually disappear with the treatment.

One medicine that was tested very thoroughly for treatment of apnea was protriptyline. This medicine has been used for many years against depression. One of its effects is to increase muscle tone, including the tone of the throat muscles. Since the problem in snoring and sleep apnea is floppy throat muscles, it was an attractive possibility that this medication might reverse apnea and snoring. Initial reports indicated that protriptyline was useful—it reduced snoring loudness and frequency, reduced the number of apnea episodes, and improved oxygen levels in the blood. However, the dosages necessary to bring about this improvement caused side effects, including difficulty in urination in men. Because of the side effects, if you and your doctor decide to try this drug for your snoring and apnea, it is important that you go to an expert in its use who will begin treating you with the proper dosage and will provide careful monitoring and dosage adjustment.

Similar to protriptyline, nicotine has a stimulating effect on muscle tone. It was thought in early investigations to be a potentially useful treatment of sleep apnea. However, subsequent investigations did not confirm its usefulness.

Progesterone has been tried. This hormone is known to stimulate breathing and is sometimes useful in patients with central sleep apnea. These are the people who stop breathing in their sleep, not because their airway is blocked but because they have a reduced drive to breathe. However, whether this treatment has any effect on snoring is not known.

The bottom line is that none of the drugs that have been tried for treatment are very useful. And very few physicians are now prescribing them for snoring or sleep apnea.

7

Allergies and Snoring

According to the National Center for Health Statistics, about one in every six people has an allergy of some kind. Some of these allergies are respiratory, causing the stuffy, runny nose; sneezing; and itchy, watery eyes of hayfever. These are the allergies that can sometimes cause or aggravate snoring. They cause swollen membranes—including the tissues of the nose and throat—and thus cause snoring. Sometimes these allergies constrict the bronchial tubes, causing the wheezing and chest tightness of asthma. Several studies have shown an increased apnea index in patients with allergic rhinitis during the pollen season.

What Causes Allergies?

Allergies can be caused by things you breathe (such as dust, some chemical fumes, animal dander, feathers, pollen, molds), by things you eat or drink (foods, drinks, medicines), or by things you touch (fabrics, plants, metals, wood, plastics, cosmetics, soaps). Most often something you breathe—something in the air—causes your nasal or throat tissues to swell, thus possibly causing snoring.

It's not always easy to find the cause of your allergies, but think about some of the most common things in the air that might be causing your particular problem: animal dander, ragweed, grass pollen, tree pollen, molds, dust. More than a third of allergy sufferers have reactions to cats and dogs, mostly cats. (Dr. Linde can't visit one of her friends because of cats in the house.) One young woman came to the St. Michael's sleep clinic with allergies and asthma. She both snored and wheezed at night at home, but her symptoms improved when she slept at her parents' house. It turned out that her symptoms were brought on by the dog that slept on her bed. Her parents had no pets.

An allergy can be caused by something at home or at work. Along with Dr. Hoffstein and his colleagues at St. Michael's, Dr. Arthur Leznoff and Dr. James S. Haight, reported in the *American Review of Respiratory Disease* on a case of a man who developed an allergy while working at a pet food processing plant. He suffered from snoring and apnea, as well as a runny nose and inflamed eyes, headaches, and a severe cough. For a full year he had found it difficult to get up in the morning because of fatigue, and he developed a tendency to fall asleep during the day. His wife said that he tended to choke in his sleep, that his sleep had become increasingly restless, and that he snored so loudly that she was forced to sleep in a separate room. He worked in an area about fifty feet away from where the pet food was mixed, and the most abundant dust in the air was guar gum powder, which was blown onto the surface of the food mixture. When he remained off work for seventeen days, his symptoms went away, including daytime sleepiness and morning fatigue, his snoring and restlessness decreased, and in the sleep lab his apnea was gone. The next day, for confirmation of the cause of his symptoms, he was challenged by inhaling guar gum powder. Within ten minutes he developed symptoms: a sneezing, runny nose, nasal obstruction, and inflamed eyes. These symptoms plus a hacking cough lasted six hours, and sleep tests that night showed that snoring and apnea had returned. When he returned to work a few days later, he began to suffer again from a cough, a runny nose, inflamed eyes, snoring, fitful sleep, and daytime sleepiness. After three weeks he quit his job and started working at a different job. All symptoms disappeared, and he got well. His only problem now is that he has to avoid eating ice cream or other foods that contain guar gum. In this case, it was possible to isolate the allergy as the cause of snoring and alleviate this man's—and his wife's—nighttime suffering.

How Do Allergies Cause Snoring?

Although allergies are very prevalent in the general population, they are not always associated with snoring. However, it is one of the things that we investigate in snoring patients who come to St. Michael's Hospital. Sometimes even if the nasal congestion from the allergy is not the primary cause of snoring, it can still be a factor that helps bring about the snoring or makes it worse. So even though your allergy might not be the biggest cause of snoring, it is something you should consider as you look for what is causing your particular problem.

Allergies cause swelling of nasal tissues and stuffiness, increased nasal airway resistance, and similar swelling of tissues in the throat, which invariably lead to difficulty in breathing through the nose, and may or may not result in snoring.

At St. Michael's, treatment of allergies with nasal decongestants, anti-inflammatory nasal steroid sprays, or antihistamines leads to decreased snoring in about 10 percent of patients. In other cases, our patients say that their breathing is better as a result of these medications, but their snoring has not diminished.

In general, allergies to inhaled particles such as pollen from ragweed, grass, and trees are more likely to cause nasal congestion and worsen snoring. Food allergies are rarely involved.

An allergist can do skin tests, but often you can determine the cause yourself by playing detective and thinking through the clues. For example, ask yourself these questions:

- Is there any timing pattern in the appearance of symptoms? Do symptoms tend to be related to pollen season in spring, summer, or fall, or to spring-cleaning? Or do symptoms occur year-round?

- Do the symptoms persist for long periods, or do they occur periodically, stopping and starting?

- Are the symptoms related to any special place, such as appearing at home but not away, or appearing only in certain rooms? Do they improve when you go on vacation away from home and work?

- Do symptoms appear when you are doing a particular type of task, such as playing with the cat, cleaning the attic, or looking at old books or papers?

Use the answers to these questions to help determine whether you have an allergy that might be affecting your snoring.

If Pollen Is the Problem

If sneezing, a stuffy, runny nose—and snoring—occur in August and September, you are probably allergic to ragweed pollen. If you have the problem in the spring, it is probably tree pollen; if in summer, it is likely grass pollen.

Here's what you can do to minimize your allergy symptoms:

- Keep windows closed at night, especially in early morning when pollen levels are highest, and whenever it's windy. Air-conditioning is the best preventive for pollen allergies.

- If you have handled machine oils or other things you are allergic to, wash your hands thoroughly and keep your hands away from your eyes.

- Many people find that taking extra vitamin C during pollen season may help. If an attack is starting, taking about 1,500 mg of vitamin C may relieve symptoms. Sometimes eating an orange, including the white inner peel, might also help.

- Avoid cigarette smoke.

- Sometimes it helps to take a very hot shower and inhale the steam, or to drink a hot beverage or have a hot cup of soup.

- If it's a seasonal pollen to which you are allergic and your symptoms are severe, you may find that the simplest solution is to take a vacation during that season—go to a place that is free of the pollen you're allergic to, such as the desert or the far northern woods, or go on a cruise. By all means, use Dr. Linde's new book, *The World's Most Intimate Cruises* (Open Road Publishing), to find a nifty place.

If Your Pet Is the Problem

One of the biggest causes of allergies is animal dander. In fact, the American Academy of Allergy and Immunology estimates that 20 to 30 percent of all allergy and asthma patients are allergic to animals, especially cats. Hayfever symptoms can be triggered by dander in the air, or by saliva from slobbering or fur licking, which can permeate the air in a dried form.

Other animals besides cats can cause allergies too, including dogs, monkeys, guinea pigs, hamsters, rabbits, and birds. Short hair, long hair, fuzz, or feathers—all can cause allergy symptoms. If you've got an allergy and you have a pet, think about whether it might be the cause. You might have to work doggedly to ferret out the culprit, but it will be worth it.

You may have to find your pet another home, or at least keep it outside, but first make sure that it is the cause. See an allergist for a few simple allergy tests that can confirm or rule out the diagnosis. Or take a vacation (without any pets)—if your problem improves after a few days and returns when you are with your pet again, it is likely the problem. Or if you have no vacation plans, you can put your pet in a kennel or with friends for a week or two while you have the house cleaned thoroughly, vacuuming rugs, drapes, and furniture a couple of times and washing down hard surfaces to get rid of hair and dander. If sniffing and sneezing—and snoring—stop, you can bet it was the cat or other pet that was causing the problem. However, if after taking these measures you still have symptoms, then something other than your pet is causing the trouble.

You May Be Allergic to Your House

Sometimes your allergy can be caused by things in your house. Here are some typical allergy-producing places to check:

- A rug may have a moldy pad.
- You may be allergic to a feather pillow, or an old dusty pillow.
- An old chair may have down cushions, or be dusty.
- There may be mold in the basement.
- There may be dust in the attic.

If you have hayfever or asthma from pollen, chances are that you are also allergic to dust. Be especially suspicious of dust if your symptoms get worse when you clean or when you turn on the heating or air-conditioning unit.

Actually, sometimes it's not fuzzy dust balls that cause the problem, but bits of insect wings and other bug parts that are in dust. Allergies can be produced by mayflies, houseflies, mites, cockroaches, and fruit flies. Nearly all dust contains insect substances. In fact, at Northwestern University Medical School, researchers found that nearly 30 percent of all hayfever and asthma patients studied were sensitive to one or more insects, and the National Institutes of Health estimate that some 10 to 15 million people are allergic to cockroaches and cockroach droppings, a problem that occurs particularly in old city buildings.

The most troublesome insect is the dust mite. In fact, some studies show that perhaps half of all allergic people in the world are allergic to dust mites. Hundreds of these insects will fit on a fingernail. Their droppings, which are frequently present in dust, are often the real cause of dust allergy. They especially like to hide out in carpets, upholstered furniture, mattresses, pillows, and stuffed toys. And they can be present even if you are an excellent housekeeper.

Mold is another allergen that is often the problem. Mold grows nearly everywhere—on bread and fruit, in grains and grasses, in hay and soil, in furniture and mattresses, in the shower, in humidifiers and air conditioners, in drip pans or gaskets of refrigerators, on cloth, paper, and leather, on old books, in damp cellars, in attics, and in barns. If a room smells musty, it's got mold. It's a particular problem in rainy, damp regions.

How to Allergy-Proof Your House

If you think an allergy might be causing your snoring, your house might be causing your allergy. Consider allergy-proofing your house. Here's how:

- Get rid of old upholstered furniture.
- Keep furnishings simple. Avoid dust-catching knickknacks.
- Get rid of drapes, shag rugs, chenille bedspreads, and old feather pillows.
- Wash bedding frequently in hot water. Cover your mattress with a breathable fabric, or replace it with a water bed.
- Use filters in your heating and air-conditioning system. If you have hot-air registers, put several layers of cheesecloth over or under the register to help filter the air passing through. You may need to hire a professional company to clean out your air ducts if you live in an older home.

- Clean heating/air-conditioning filters frequently. Consider a high efficiency particulate air (HEPA) filter for your furnace and air-conditioning unit.
- Make sure the clothes dryer is vented to the outside.
- Try to have someone else do the housecleaning. Make sure the cleaners clean under and behind furniture, over the tops of doors and window frames, and that they use a cloth rather than a feather duster.
- Vacuuming should be done frequently and should include furniture as well as carpets.
- Do not allow tobacco smoke or kerosene or oil burners in your house.
- During pollen season, use central air-conditioning to decrease the amount of pollen entering your home, or keep bedroom windows closed.
- Store seldom-used things in plastic bags.
- Discourage cockroaches by keeping the attic ventilated, keeping food off countertops, and taking garbage out every evening.
- Get rid of old furniture, mattresses, books, or other materials that seem to be moldy.
- If mold is a problem, use a dehumidifier, or paint walls with a mold inhibitor. Allow adequate ventilation of rooms and storage areas. Take care that shoes, gloves, and suitcases are not allowed to become moldy.
- Use antimold tile cleaner or a solution of bleach and water to clean the shower. Wash the shower curtain frequently. Clean mold-collecting places such as refrigerator pans frequently and use a germicide. Don't overwater plants—it encourages mold to form on the soil.

Organic Solvents

Dr. Jan Ulfberg at Avesta Hospital, Dr. Christer Edling at the University Hospital in Uppsala, and others in Sweden suspected that exposure to organic solvents could also be a cause of sleep-disordered breathing. They investigated whether there was a higher prevalence of sleep apnea among people with occupational exposure to organic solvents than among their neighbors. They found that people with apnea and snoring living in one area had indeed been exposed more often to organic solvents, and they found almost a twofold increase in sleep-disordered breathing in people who were exposed for entire workdays. Others had reported earlier that organic solvents could cause apnea (organic solvents are central nervous system depressants), but this was the first time that such solvents had been shown to cause snoring. It is something to look out for.

Medications to Take

There are many medications, both prescription and over-the-counter, available to help with allergies. Antihistamine tablets work to alleviate runny nose, watery eyes, and sneezing. Taken when you go to bed, they will help shrink nasal tissues and make it easier for you to breathe. Even if you use over-the-counter antihistamines, consult with your physician to be sure that you use only an antihistamine that does not depress the central nervous system, or make you sleepy, spacey, or depressed. Some antihistamines act just like tranquilizers and sleeping pills: they deepen sleep and cause greater relaxation of airway tissues, which can aggravate snoring. Ask your doctor about taking a nonsedating antihistamine. Also check with your doctor and pharmacist about other medicines that you are taking, since they sometimes interact with antihistamines and cause side effects. With some antihistamines, you should not eat grapefruit or drink grapefruit juice because higher levels of the antihistamine can be produced in the body. And remember, if you take an antihistamine, you should not drink alcohol.

In men with prostate problems, some antihistamines may aggravate the problem. Dr. Hoffstein once prescribed an antihistamine to a friend who was a loud snorer. The treatment worked, but after three weeks the friend landed in the doctor's office complaining of urinary problems. Investigation revealed that he had an infection of the prostate. Prompt discontinuation of the antihistamine resolved the problem. They are still friends.

There are nose sprays that may be helpful also, but all nose sprays are not alike. *Corticosteroid sprays,* available only by prescription, help relieve congestion from inflammation and nasal polyps. They are used daily, not sporadically, and they take at least several days to become fully effective. They sometimes leave an unpleasant taste in the mouth. They are effective, but do not use them more often than your doctor recommends. A *nonsteroid nasal spray* called cromolyn sodium, available over the counter as Nasalcrom, is effective to prevent sneezing and itchy, runny nose. It is used at least four times a day, starting four to six weeks before the start of allergy season. Instead of blocking histamine after its release, it prevents cells from reacting to things you are allergic to. There are also *over-the-counter decongestants* such as Afrin, Dristan, Neo-Synephrine, Nostril, and Otrivin, which are primarily indicated for congestion due to colds, but are sometimes used for nasal allergies. They work partly by shrinking swollen membranes, which can help open nasal passages. But they should not be used constantly, since they can become habit-forming, cause rebound congestion, and lead to what doctors call "nose spray addiction," and can also aggravate high blood pressure or an irregular heartbeat. Simple sprays that can be used as needed without causing problems are the several brands of over-the-counter salt-water sprays. These will relieve mild congestion, loosen mucus, and prevent crusting. (You can make your own salt-water spray with boiled water and salt. Make a fresh supply weekly.) At St. Michael's, a simple hydrating agent such as Secaris gel or salt solution is used for people with nasal dryness. This sometimes helps decrease snoring. If you have problems with insomnia, be sure to avoid nasal sprays that contain phenylpropanolamine (PPA) or pseudoephedrine, or herbal remedies containing ephedra, all of which can cause anxiety or insomnia or raise blood pressure.

Several homeopathic and herbal preparations are also marketed for allergies. Several are over-the-counter preparations mainly used to relieve itchy eyes caused by allergies but that also help clear nasal congestion.

There are also some new drugs now being developed that act on the substances in the body that cause inflammation, but do not cause drowsiness and do not contain steroids. There are also some new anti-inflammatory sprays being developed. Watch for them as they become available and discuss with your doctor whether to use them.

Before you take any allergy medication, you should discuss it with your doctor. There may be reasons you should not take a certain medication. One medication may interact with another, or one may be better than another in your particular case. Your pharmacist should also be told of all the various medications you are taking in order to check for interactions or conflicts. It is recommended that people with heart disease or over age 60 should not take the antihistamine Hismanal or Seldane, nor should patients with abnormal heart rhythms since it potentiates the abnormal rhythms. Seldane has been taken off the market. Hismanal should also not be taken by people taking certain high blood pressure drugs or certain antibiotics or antidepressants. Men with prostatic hypertrophy leading to urinary obstruction should not take the antihistamines Chlortrimeton or Dimetane, and people with high blood pressure should not take antihistamines or decongestants that contain ephedrine or pseudoephedrine, which could raise blood pressure. Especially helpful to the person who snores or who has apnea are the antihistamines that do not depress the central nervous system and do not (usually) cause drowsiness, such as Allegra, Claritin, and Zyrtec. However, be careful if there is a "D" after the name (e.g., Allegra-D). This means that a decongestant has been added and it could be pseudoephedrine, which could keep you awake or cause other side effects.

If other treatments have not worked, you may also want to discuss with an allergist whether to take allergy shots. These are time-consuming, but have been shown to be effective in many people who have pollen, dust, or cat allergies.

8

Snore Balls and Other Simple Solutions

George Catlin, an artist and a lawyer who for decades studied the customs of American Indians, wrote a book based on his experiences that was published back in 1872 by our same publisher—John Wiley & Sons. In the book, titled *The Breath of Life,* he attributed the good health of Native Americans to the fact that they are taught from an early age to sleep with the mouth shut and to breathe through the nose. Catlin may also have been one of the first persons to recognize the excessive daytime sleepiness that often is the fate of habitual snorers. "That man knows not the pleasure of sleep," he wrote. "He rises in the morning more fatigued than when he retired to rest."

If you have eliminated smoking, heavy drinking, and sleeping pills from your life, you have gotten your weight to a recommended level, and you have checked for allergies and other medical conditions that might be causing your snoring and have corrected them, then your next step might be to try a few simple remedies that have helped some snorers in the past.

In this chapter we describe some home remedies and unconventional techniques that have been tried to alleviate snoring and sleep apnea. There is no rigorous scientific evidence that these techniques work in many snorers. They may work in some. The decision regarding using any of these techniques should be made based on the risk-benefit ratio, that is, after carefully considering the balance between the possible side effects and the chance of success. There is usually no harm in trying a remedy whose risk is very low, even if the chance of success is also low. We give our recommendation after the description of each treatment. These remedies probably won't cure your snoring, but some of them may help reduce its severity. If you decide to try any of them, ask your bedpartner to check whether the remedy has made a difference in your particular case.

Shut Your Mouth

Doing as the Indians and learning to breathe through your nose while you sleep is one of the simplest remedies and can be quite helpful.

In fact, Catlin's book regarding the benefits of breathing through the nose was so popular that the next edition of his book was titled *Shut Your Mouth and Save Your Life.*

Not long after publication of the books, there was a flurry of patented inventions of appliances designed to keep the mouth shut by forced closure. There is a collection of them in the U.S. Patent Office archives and library. Some of them are quite ingenious in their design. One of the earliest was a cap with a strap that fit under the chin. Another, patented in 1899, was a "mouth button" that had two sections of soft material held together by a screw. One section fit between the front teeth and the inner surface of the lips, and the other fit against the outer surface of the lips. A device patented in 1926 consisted of a remarkable combination of chin and head straps tightened in several places.

A simpler way to keep the mouth shut that works for some people is to lie on one side and simply prop your fist gently under your chin. Or if your nose seems a little stuffy, you can prop your thumb under your chin and with your middle finger push your nose up slightly to help open the passageway. Or you can prop the pillow under your chin to hold your mouth shut. After a few nights you will automatically assume such a position, and believe it or not, it isn't uncomfortable. These techniques are risk-free and you can try them.

Pillows

Many people find that sleeping in an elevated position helps, and this has been confirmed by several studies, mainly of patients with sleep apnea who snored. For example, Dr. Douglas McEvoy and colleagues in Australia found that sleeping in a sitting position at a 60 degree angle

KEEPING YOUR MOUTH SHUT

In 1989 an interesting exchange of letters between Canadian physicians was published in the *Canadian Medical Association Journal* dealing with methods of keeping the mouth closed. Dr. Michael Lattey, of Vancouver, British Columbia, suggested placing a small piece of micropore tape over the lips to force the snorer to breathe through the nose. Another physician said he had begun experimenting with tape and gave these suggestions: "Fold a narrow pull tab over at each end of the tape. Close the lips firmly before applying the tape. Transpore tape allows more air transfer and is relatively easy to remove. Adhesive tape remover is useful for any residue on the skin."

He cautioned against taping the mouth closed if there is any possibility of sleep apnea, other breathing difficulties, or nasal obstruction.

Another doctor joined the discussion and said it wouldn't work for him or his wife. He had a mustache and beard so the tape wouldn't stick, and she snored through her nose. His suggested solution was rather desperate: "a clothespin on the nose, a large safety pin to seal the lips and a tracheotomy." He added: "If Lattey would have hope that he could find a more humane solution and would like to study my wife's case, I invite him to spend one or more nights in bed with her. I'll vacate my privileged sleeping site but will insist that he have more rectitude to such a degree that he will with certainty be capable of combining propriety and propinquity."

reduces the number of apnea episodes by about 60 percent because it makes the upper airways less collapsible.

Some people buy special pillows to elevate the head at an angle, or you can simply put a wedge under a pillow or sleep on two pillows. But the best way to sleep is not to bend your neck. Elevate the bed instead. Tilting the bed takes pressure off the diaphragm and eases breathing. Pillows that make you bend at the neck can add to obstructed breathing.

There are also pillows designed to keep you from sleeping with your head back by forcing your head to the side. One of the earliest such pillows was designed by Peter Sandler (and is called the Sandler pillow). It has an indentation for the head, with a rod in the middle of the indentation that forces you to turn your head to the side. Drs.

Daniel Brunner and Jürg Schwander, of Zurich, Switzerland, studied a pillow designed in Switzerland to prevent sleeping on the back. Ten people learned to use the pillow at home, then were tested in the sleep lab, using a normal pillow one night and the new pillow another night. Their snoring was shown to be reduced from 41 percent to 25 percent of their total sleep time. The number of episodes of sleep apnea was also reduced significantly.

Get Off Your Back

A patient went to the doctor with bruises all over his legs. Could it be a blood disorder causing bleeding under the skin? Could it be a side effect of a blood-thinning medication? Neither. Careful interviewing determined that his wife was kicking him dozens of times throughout the night in an effort to make him turn over. "Honey, turn over—you're snoring" wasn't working anymore, and he was too heavy to shove, so she had resorted to more drastic measures: a few swift kicks.

Almost universally, snoring occurs more often when people sleep on the back. Not sleeping on the back really can make a difference in many people. At St. Michael's, many patients who come in for snoring problems are benefited from this simple change in sleeping position. The reason: sleeping on the side helps keep the mouth closed, as gravity is not pulling the jaw open, and nasal breathing is helped by the reflex that opens one nasal passage when you sleep on the other one.

Here are a number of simple ways to keep from sleeping on your back:

- Try one of the special pillows we described, or wedge a pillow or a teddy bear against your back to keep you from turning over.
- Elevate your head, especially if you are overweight. You can do this by placing a wedge from a medical supply store under the mattress or by putting blocks (usually 6-inch ones are recommended) under the head of the bed.
- Try using snore balls. Put three tennis balls in a sock and sew them onto the back of your pajamas. The name "snore balls" was coined by some sleep experts, possibly after being up all night in the sleep lab. We don't know why three balls are used, or why golf balls aren't used, only that three tennis balls are

what always seems to be recommended. Actually just about any-thing will work: three marbles in a pouch, an empty spool of thread in a sock, whatever. Just so long as whenever you turn over on your back, the tennis balls or marbles or whatever poke you and you wake up enough to turn onto your side. Dr. Ros-alind Cartwright, director of the sleep disorders center at Rush-Presbyterian–St. Luke's Medical Center in Chicago, invented the Sleep Position Monitor, a little blue box worn on the chest that beeps if the sleeper flips on the back. Dr. Cartwright says that the beeper acts as a training device and can actually teach people not to sleep on the back.

These changes in sleeping position can help both snoring and ap-nea. Recently Dr. Alister McKenzie and a team of researchers at the sleep disorders unit of Repatriation General Hospital in Adelaide, Aus-tralia, did a series of studies of patients who had obstructive sleep ap-nea. When the upper body was elevated 30 degrees or when the patient slept on the side, the number of apnea events was decreased.

While these positional changes will help many people, some people will snore in any position. The only way to determine whether posi-tional changes will work for you is to try them. There is no risk and it might help.

Nasal Dilators

After Catlin's observation regarding the importance of "shutting your mouth," physicians began to notice how nighttime nasal obstruction and mouth breathing could affect daytime performance. In 1889 Dr. D. Guye of Amsterdam described patients with daytime fatigue and in-ability to concentrate, and even came up with a name for their condi-tion: *aprosexia nasalis.* In 1892 Dr. Louis Cline described a locomotive engineer who suffered from severe nasal obstruction night and day and whose daytime sleepiness was so bad he would fall asleep on the job. Dr. Cline said that on awakening, the engineer "could not tell where he was or what station he had passed last . . . or whether he had orders to run or not." Following surgery to correct his nasal obstruction, all his symptoms disappeared.

In 1905 Dr. A. Francis described a mechanical nasal dilator that fits inside the nose, which was used for many years to reduce nasal resistance. More recently a device made of flexible plastic, called a Nozovent, was developed in Sweden, that is inserted into the nose and uses an outward springboard action to dilate the nostrils. Between 1988 and 1994 there were studies in Sweden and Japan showing that Nozovent improved nasal breathing and reduced snoring and apnea. Drs. Steen Löth and the inventor Björn Petruson, of the University of Göteborg, did a study of forty-two men who were heavy snorers and found that using the Nozovent device decreased snoring and morning tiredness. About 60 percent of the patients continued to use the device at six months. Others have found less positive results—the patient's breathing is easier, but snoring may or may not be reduced.

Another device used on the inside of the nostrils is Breathe-With-EEZ, a flexible stainless steel coil that is inserted into each nostril.

Some people have trouble with these devices coming out at night. If you try these devices and find them uncomfortable, it sometimes helps to insert them about ten minutes before you go to bed to get used to them.

Another type of nasal dilator is Breathe Right nasal strip. This device uses the technique of putting tape on the outside of the nose to widen the nasal openings and improve air intake. It was developed by a man with a deviated septum to help his own breathing problem and later was used by football players to improve their breathing. It was adapted in 1993 for medical use. Now it's used by many athletes and by people with nasal congestion and/or snoring problems. The Breathe Right device consists of an adhesive strip with a plastic backbone. The strip is bent over the bridge of the nose, and the ends applied to the soft tissue at the flare of each nostril. The plastic strip attempts to straighten and this action lifts the sides of the nose, pulling apart the nasal openings, thus widening the nasal passages and making it easier to breathe. In the *Ear, Nose, and Throat Journal*, Dr. Martin B. Scharf of the Center for Research in Sleep Disorders at Mercy Hospital in Cincinnati reported that in a study of twenty snorers, approximately three out of four experienced either easier breathing, quieter snoring, better sleep quality, or less daytime sleepiness after using the strips. Another study, by Drs. Jan Ulfberg of the Avesta Hospital in Sweden and Gus Fenton of the Breathe Right manufacturing company, reported about half of thirty-two snorers snored less and had less daytime sleepiness with the nasal strips. However, other studies did not show beneficial effects.

These strips and the other devices can be purchased in most drugstores or grocery stores, or in sporting goods stores. It can sometimes take a week to ten days of using them to successfully retrain yourself to breathe through your nose and close your mouth while you sleep. They may or may not eliminate your snoring, but some people have found they reduce snoring considerably. As always, you need to decide for yourself. There is no risk or serious side effect.

Open and Soothe the Nose and Throat

Whatever you can do to lessen vibrations in the nose and throat or to reduce irritation or obstruction and open the airways will help prevent snoring. There are a number of things that you might wish to try. Again, these things work in some people but not in others. If you decide to try them, you need to determine for yourself with as objective an attitude as possible whether they work for you.

Increasing the Humidity in Your Bedroom

Dry air irritates nasal and throat passages, causing them to be inflamed. This further narrows the airways and facilitates snoring. Humidifying the air often reduces dry-air irritation and helps prevent inflammation, thus reducing snoring in some people. Sitting in a closed bathroom and breathing the steam from a hot shower or using a vaporizer can also help clear airways.

Homeopathic Products

Some of the newest things on the market are pills to help stop snoring. These pills mostly use enzymes and herbs to break up mucus and help clear airways. One brand is SnoreStop. It is an over-the-counter formula whose ingredients, in a very diluted solution, are nux vomica (Quaker buttons), ephedra (Mormon tea), histaminum hydrochloride (from an amino acid), *Teucrium marum* (cat-thyme), *Hydrastis canadensis* (goldenseal), *Atropa belladonna* (belladonna berries), and kali bichromicum (bichromate of potash). The various individual ingredients work to reduce snoring by reducing swelling, firming and shrinking tissues in the nose and throat, alleviating sinus congestion and drainage, and relieving nasal congestion from allergies. You take one or two tablets at bedtime, letting them dissolve. When steady improvement is noticed, the dosage can be reduced to every other day, and gradually decreased. SnoreStop was tested in one hundred persons in Portland, Oregon, who snored but did not have apnea. There was significant, but not complete, reduction in snoring in those treated compared to those receiving a placebo pill. Studies on these products have not been published in well-known medical journals; however, there are some snorers who say that their snoring is reduced or eliminated when using these remedies.

Nose Drops and Sprays

Corticosteroid or decongestant nose drops or sprays for allergies and colds, whether obtained by prescription or over the counter, may relieve snoring, particularly during the allergy season or when you have a cold and cannot breathe through your stuffy nose. However, none of them are recommended for long-term regular use to relieve snoring. There are a number of brands of over-the-counter salt-water sprays that can be used as needed to relieve nasal congestion, loosen mucus, and help prevent crusting. Also available are several brands of nose drops made of root, herb, and flower extracts that are designed to open the airways to help counteract snoring.

The research team at St. Michael's Hospital decided to try to find some way to reduce the vibrations that cause snoring, and thought of perhaps reducing turbulent airflow by coating the nose and throat passages with a friction-reducing agent. They tested a preparation called Sonarite that was derived from a combination of lecithin and mineral oil. When used as nose drops, the thin oil adhered to the nose and throat tissues and functioned as a lubricating agent. The results showed a reduction in the number of snores per hour and snoring loudness. However, mineral oil can sometimes get into the lungs and cause pneumonia. A new solution is being tested that does not contain mineral oil. In fact, Dr. Michael Fitzpatrick and colleagues of the University of Saskatchewan in Saskatoon, Canada, reported at the annual meeting of the Association of Professional Sleep Societies in 1997 that using a modified preparation of Sonarite that does not contain mineral oil reduced the number of episodes of apnea and hypopnea from twenty-five per hour during the night when a placebo was used to fourteen per hour during the night when Sonarite was used. However, this product is still experimental, there are no long-term studies of it, and it is only available as part of a research study.

Nutritional Aids

Some snorers try nutritional aids. There are no published scientific studies on their use, and the evidence for their beneficial effects is what scientists call "anecdotal." Some of them are harmless and you may want to try them to see if they work for you. Others may be associated with side effects and we do not recommend them.

- Try drinking a hot liquid before you go to bed. This can often keep your nose and throat passages free of congestion, at least for a while.

- For years grandmothers advised a tablespoon of honey in hot water before bedtime to clear nasal congestion from a stuffy or runny nose. Others have recommended chewing honeycomb to keep the nose dry and open. Apple cider vinegar has also been recommended for a stuffy nose. The vinegar is mixed in water, sometimes with honey, and drunk before bed to get rid of excess mucus.

- Eat citrus fruits for their vitamin C and bioflavonoids. Another good home remedy for stuffy nose is to eat a fresh orange, including the white stuff inside the skin; or to grind a lemon or orange in the garbage disposal and bend over it and deeply breathe in the aroma for several minutes. Taking a vitamin C supplement will often help clear a stuffy nose due to an allergy or a cold.

- Drink herbal teas, available at health food stores. Breathe Easy, for example, is a tea formulated to temporarily restore freer breathing through the nose. It is made up of pseudoephedrine in ma huang (*Ephedra sinica*), plus peppermint leaf, licorice root, fennel seed, eucalyptus leaf, pleurisy root, calendula flower, and ginger. (However, you should not use this or other forms of pseudoephedrine if you have high blood pressure.)

- L-tryptophan, a nutritional supplement, was used in 1983 by Dr. Helmut Schmidt, of Ohio State University at Columbus, in a study of fifteen patients with sleep apnea. An average dose of

2,500 mg was given at bedtime. There was significant improvement in patients with obstructive sleep apnea, but not with central sleep apnea. L-tryptophan was banned by the FDA in the United States because of side effects from batches that were contaminated in manufacture several years ago and is not currently available. This study hasn't been confirmed yet, and further research is needed to determine the role of this agent. We do not recommend that you use L-tryptophan without consulting your doctor.

Simple Exercises

Snoring experts today do not believe that throat and jaw muscle exercises, such as gum chewing or jaw clenching, are effective in combating snoring. However, a British physician, Dr. Harvey Flack, tested various exercises and concluded that exercises that tense the muscles to keep the mouth closed helped eliminate mouth breathing. He instructed people to hold something between the teeth for ten minutes before going to bed. After four or five minutes, usually the jaw muscles began to ache. But if the exercises were done for many hours, the muscle tone increased, he claimed. Dr. Flack also described an exercise to strengthen the muscles that hold the lower jaw and tongue forward. This resistance exercise consisted of pushing the finger against the front of the chin while pushing back against the finger with the jaw. Another early proponent of exercises recommended saying "ah" over and over to tense certain throat muscles, and another recommended chewing large chunks of (sugar-free) bubble gum to strengthen jaw muscles.

Very little work has been done on exercises, and few snoring experts believe that they will work. However, Dr. Martin Scharf of Mercy Hospital in Cincinnati decided to investigate the possibility. Working with fifteen volunteers who snored but did not have apnea, he had their bedpartners tape-record their snoring for two consecutive nights before and after a month of three exercises. The first exercise involved holding a pencil between the teeth and bearing down for five minutes. For the second exercise, the elbows were propped on a table and for three minutes the fingers were pressed on the front of the lower jaw while the lower jaw pushed against the fingers. The third exercise was to press the tongue against the lower teeth for three to four minutes.

Five volunteers said the exercises were too much trouble so they didn't continue, five said their snoring stopped or was dramatically improved, and five were not sure whether the snoring improved. None of these exercises to tighten tongue and jaw muscles have since been studied. However, since there is no risk to the exercises, there is no harm in trying them.

Behavior Modification

Sometimes you can help combat snoring by establishing new habits—not sleeping on your back, breathing lightly and calmly instead of forcefully, keeping your mouth closed as you go to sleep. Here are some other remedies that have been tried.

- **Electrical stimulators.** These devices operate on a different principle than any of the other remedies described so far. One of the first devices was described in 1984 by an Australian inventor, Anthony Dowling, who obtained a patent for a miniature electronic device worn in the outer ear. When the microphone sensed a snoring sound, the audio generator would awaken the snorer by emitting a loud sound. The most popular electronic device is the SnoreStopper. Worn around the arm, it senses snoring sounds and then sends an electrical impulse which feels like a sting. This causes an arousal and hopefully stops snoring. Another device is worn as a wristwatch, and another electrically stimulates muscles of the tongue, causing the tongue muscles to contract and thus open the airway. Although these devices seemed promising in the initial studies, subsequent studies have not demonstrated the usefulness of electrical stimulation for treatment of snoring or apnea. At this time we do not recommend them, although the studies of electrical stimulators are still ongoing.
- **Distraction techniques.** Since snoring occurs especially in the deep stages of sleep, one of the techniques of counteracting it is to provide some stimulus to prevent the snorer from going into the deeper stages of sleep. This usually involves some kinder, gentler alternatives to kicking or shoving your bedpartner. Some

of those techniques are musical pillows or devices that generate the sound of waves or other "quiet noise."

- **Hypnosis.** If your snoring is mostly due to a habit of sleeping on your back or breathing with your mouth open, then hypnosis may be able to help you break those habits, learning instead to sleep on your side, keep your mouth shut, and breathe through your nose. Talk to a professional about the possibilities. Or try it yourself. Each night as you go to sleep, quietly say, "I will close my mouth and breathe calmly through my nose. I will close my mouth and breathe calmly through my nose." You can also try to mentally program yourself as you go to sleep to sleep on your side rather than on your back.

- **Progressive relaxation.** Some people have found it helpful to practice progressive relaxation in bed before going to sleep. This technique encourages sleepers to breathe in a more relaxed manner and decreases the intensity of the airflow. It consists of tightening different muscle groups in the body and then letting go to learn the feeling of relaxation.

- **Other relaxation techniques.** People often report that when they go to sleep tired or stressed, they snore more. Use tai chi, deep breathing, or any relaxation technique that works for you. Try eliminating serious stress and overtiredness from your life, and try relaxing before bedtime to let go of stress. There are no risks to relaxation techniques, so it is okay to try them.

Keep Working on the Basic Causes

Remember, the simple remedies described in this chapter have not received controlled trials. They are all only aids that may help some snorers.

If these techniques do not help your snoring, do not be disappointed. Remember that there are simple proven techniques to stop your snoring—weight loss and avoidance of alcohol, for example—that will work if you adhere to them. And if they fail, there are other techniques that may work for you, which you will learn about in the remaining chapters.

9

Serious Help from CPAP and Oral Appliances

If you have eliminated cigarettes, alcohol, sleeping pills, and tranquilizers from your daily lifestyle, if you have gotten your weight to normal, if you have stopped sleeping on your back, and if you have tried the over-the-counter remedies and other simple aids we have described, and you still have a problem, then you probably should seek professional help.

In fact, you should *always* see your family physician or a sleep specialist under the following conditions:

- If snoring is severe
- If you have been observed to stop breathing in your sleep
- If you are dragging with fatigue or are excessively sleepy during the day
- If you have tried the steps we outlined in the previous chapters but still have trouble with snoring
- If in addition to snoring, you are overweight or have high blood pressure or heart disease

Your doctor or sleep specialist will be able to determine what treatments are best for you and whether you need to take more steps than those we have already described. This chapter will outline two of the modern medical treatments available to you through professional channels: continuous positive airway pressure (CPAP) and oral appliances.

Continuous Positive Airway Pressure

Only fifteen years ago or so, treatment for snoring and sleep apnea was very limited. You could get off cigarettes, alcohol, and sleeping pills, lose weight, and sleep on your side—and indeed all of those things help—or if you had sleep apnea, you could have a surgical procedure called a tracheotomy. This operation involved making a small hole in the windpipe, just below the Adam's apple. In people with sleep apnea, this operation bypassed their obstruction and allowed them to breathe at night. The operation, although successful in relieving sleep apnea, is cosmetically troublesome to patients, requires regular maintenance of the tracheotomy site in order to minimize potential complications, and is very seldom performed today.

With the development of the CPAP machine, treatment options improved for people with snoring and apnea too serious to be cured by lifestyle changes.

The CPAP system was devised in 1981 by Dr. Colin Sullivan, of Sydney, Australia, who originally described it in five patients. The name *CPAP* stands for "continuous positive airway pressure." The system involves the patient wearing a mask that fits over the nose and forms an airtight seal. A hose connects the mask to a small portable pump that blows a steady stream of air into the throat during sleep. This holds the airway open so the patient can breathe and sleep normally. The machine acts as a pneumatic splint, blasting the airway open with a stream of air. It's like a vacuum cleaner in reverse. The air pressure is adjusted so that it is just enough to prevent the throat from collapsing during sleep. The worse the snoring or apnea, or the fatter the neck of an obese person, the higher the pressure needed.

The CPAP machine has revolutionized the treatment of sleep apnea as well as serious snoring; in fact, the CPAP machine virtually abolishes snoring.

How Does It Work?

Snoring, as you recall, happens because the airway is narrowed and the airway walls are floppy; apnea goes one step further and the airway closes completely. Anything that abolishes apnea will also abolish snoring (but not necessarily the other way around). Usually higher pressures are required to abolish apnea than to abolish snoring.

In 1983 Drs. Richard Berry and A. Jay Block, of the University of Florida and the Veterans Administration Medical Center in Gainesville, tested the CPAP device in nine snorers and found that it almost completely eliminated snoring, reducing the average number of snores per night from 1,015 to 23.

To date, more than one hundred studies have confirmed its effectiveness. At this point in medical progress, CPAP is the most widely accepted and most common medical treatment for sleep apnea and the most guaranteed way to stop snoring. It is almost 100 percent successful, but it's also cumbersome and many patients cannot tolerate it.

Patient acceptance of the CPAP machine is a problem. Despite its effectiveness, at follow-up carried out between two and forty-eight months after starting CPAP, 10 to 50 percent of patients (depending on the study reported) had stopped using it.

How to Use It

Because of the discomfort in using the CPAP appliance, many snorers decline to use it, unless they have apnea and believe that medically they need to use it. In fact, Drs. Hellmuth Rauscher, Dieter Formanek, and Hartmut Zwick of Vienna offered the device to fifty-nine snorers who had snoring but did not have apnea. All complained of excessive daytime sleepiness because of their snoring, but only eleven were even willing to try the device.

Part of the problem is that the CPAP machine is uncomfortable. Most of the discomfort is due to the mask and the attachments that hold the mask against the face. In addition, its cool, dry air can affect the nose in several ways, sometimes causing increased production of mucus, sometimes causing swelling and congestion, sometimes both. If tissue swelling closes the openings of the sinuses, sinus pain and headache can also occur, or sometimes a sinus infection. A dry, irritated nose is also more likely to bleed, and the dry air in the throat can cause a burning sensation. This side effect is minimized by the use of a warm-air humidifier.

Other side effects that sometimes occur include skin irritation, abdominal bloating, sore eyes, dry mouth, and claustrophobia. Because of the benefits, many snorers agree to try CPAP but because of so many side effects, many give up after a while. It seems highly unlikely that CPAP will ever enjoy the same success in the treatment of snoring as it does in the treatment of sleep apnea, perhaps because the person with sleep apnea is more aware of the medical need to treat apnea or is more symptomatic. Patients with significant sleep apnea derive much more benefit from using the CPAP machine than do simple snorers.

Probably the best way to increase the likelihood that you'll be able to comply with using a CPAP is to reduce the discomfort and side effects. There are several ways to do this. In one study, Drs. Stephen Sheldon and Ann Reetz, of the Sleep Disorders Center at Grant Hospital in Chicago, used Breathe Right nasal strips on the noses of patients to increase the nasal airway when they had problems with CPAP. The patients applied the nasal strips at bedtime just before beginning the CPAP, wearing the strip under the CPAP mask. Nasal side effects were relieved in one day, and compliance increased.

Sometimes it is helpful in counteracting the side effect of nasal congestion to humidify the room. But this is now seldom necessary, since most CPAP blowers are equipped with humidifiers. You can also use nasal decongestants or antihistamines to help with congestion. A nasal decongestant spray may help by decreasing swelling; however, there may be a rebound effect if used nightly, and it may then cause nasal stuffiness. Sometimes a nasal steroid spray will help by decreasing the swelling and irritation of the nasal passages. Or you may wish to lubricate the nasal passages with a nasal lubricant. In patients with perennial rhinitis, a spray containing ipratropium bromide will help. Sometimes it helps to simply use a salt water nasal spray or flush the nostrils with an over-the-counter or homemade salt solution during the day and at bedtime. Having the respiratory technologist adjust the air pressure to the lowest value needed to abolish snoring can also make a difference.

If the bedroom is cool, tuck the CPAP tubing under the covers to warm the air. If your face is irritated, using a different mask may help, or alternating between two. There are now new masks made of nonirritating material that fit snugly against the face without exerting any pressure. Skin moisturizers may also help.

Once you and your physician have decided you should try CPAP, you will need to be fitted for a mask and headgear that are comfortable for you and that provide a good seal for air pressure to build up. The mask is worn over your nose and held in place by adjustable straps. Headgear straps are adjusted to be tight enough for a good fit in all sleeping positions, but not so tight as to be uncomfortable. The hose should be no more than twelve feet long. There are now many masks on the market. Some are made out of a soft gel-like material that molds

SERIOUS HELP FROM CPAP AND ORAL APPLIANCES • 119

more easily to the face and may be more comfortable. Others have a bubble that can also adapt to the contours of the face. It's okay, by the way, to use a mask made by one company with a CPAP machine made by another. It is also possible to have masks custom-made. Some masks are made especially for mustache and beard wearers. If you are allergic to the usual silicone material, you can get a mask made from rubber or vinyl.

Some patients may prefer a full face mask instead of a nasal mask. It fits along the outside of the face and may be more comfortable because it causes less pressure on the skin and has fewer leaks that can irritate the eyes. Other patients get relief using nasal pillows, which look like small plugs and fit under the nostrils.

Before deciding on a mask, try it with a CPAP machine and turn your head from side to side in different sleeping positions.

The National Center on Sleep Disorders Research of the National Institutes of Health recommends follow-up after the first month of CPAP use. The follow-up should include checking the status of equipment, assessing patient symptoms and adherence, and assessing the status of coexisting conditions such as high blood pressure. If you have achieved significant weight loss, the CPAP pressure may need to be lowered, and if your snoring has continued, the pressure may need to be increased. According to a report given at the meeting of the Associated Professional Sleep Societies in San Francisco in 1997, the CPAP pressure requirements seem to decrease within two weeks of starting the treatment, so your CPAP specialist can often lower your pressure after two weeks and make the treatment much more comfortable.

CPAP is still the mainstay of apnea treatment, and constant advances are being made in the design of the mask, headgear, and blowers. Humidification of air going into nasal passages is now almost universal on all machines. Another useful feature that has improved acceptance is "ramping": the air pressure is started low and then gradually increased to the full prescribed pressure. For example, if you set the ramp time at 20, it will take twenty minutes for the pressure to reach the prescribed value. This will allow you to fall asleep more easily because you will not be irritated by high pressure.

Machine Options

Probably the two most important advances in the design of the CPAP machine are bilevel pressure and automatic setting of the pressure. Bilevel pressure machines, called BiPAP, allow you to set different pressures for inhalation and exhalation. Setting lower pressure for exhalation makes the system much more comfortable because you do not have to breathe out against a strong airflow. New machines feature an automatic setting that allows the pressure to be automatically adjusted by a special device inside the machine that senses snoring or apnea. These machines are called SmartPAP, DPAP, or Autoset, depending on the manufacturer, and are now being evaluated and tested.

CPAPs are not cheap—they cost from $1,000 to $3,000—but as one sleep researcher has said, "It's cheaper than divorce." You can also rent one for two or three months to see how it works for you before purchasing it. In fact, you may want to test more than one device and see which one suits you the best. Health insurance plans will usually cover some of the costs of a CPAP.

If you have questions about different machines or mask options, consult with your physician or a sleep center, or contact the American Sleep Apnea Association (see Appendix B). Here are some of the questions you may want to ask when you are deciding about any CPAP machine:

- What effect will it have on your lifestyle, such as travel plans?
- What happens if you try it and it's not right for you?
- How often will there be follow-ups?
- What effects will it likely have on your health?
- Do you have any health conditions that would make the CPAP inappropriate for you?
- What if the machine needs repairs or adjustments, or you have side effects of any kind?
- What is required for maintenance?
- What special features or advantages does one machine have over other models you should be considering?

Effects of Using CPAP

How do you know if your CPAP is working? You will wake up refreshed and will be more alert and energetic during the day, and your bedpartner will no longer complain about your snoring. Most patients experience immediate improvement, frequently after just a few nights of using a CPAP machine. Some say they had forgotten what it felt like to feel good. Others say that CPAP has changed their life, giving them back their days as well as their nights.

Some long-term effects of CPAP in preventing the complications due to sleep apnea, such as high blood pressure and predisposition to strokes and heart attacks, are not yet known. However, short-term effects of sleep apnea on blood pressure have been studied extensively. For example, Drs. M. MacNaughton and R. Pierce of the Heidelberg Repatriation Hospital in Melbourne, Australia, found that after ten days of treatment with CPAP, patients with high blood pressure and sleep apnea had blood pressure reduced from 139/81 to 130/76. Dr. Donald Silverberg and colleagues, of the Sourasky Tel Aviv Medical Center, reviewed ten recent studies of the effect of treatment of sleep apnea with CPAP on blood pressure and found that in nine of the studies, the treatment of sleep apnea was also associated with reduced blood pressure. We still can't say, however, that CPAP definitely reduces blood pressure—not all investigators and studies agree. However, overall, most of the studies indicate that sleep apnea has an independent association with blood pressure, and therefore it is logical to expect that treatment of apnea in patients with high blood pressure would also help control high blood pressure.

One review of patients with moderate to severe apnea, by Dr. Yiang He and colleagues at the University of Manitoba, found that the death rate of patients treated with CPAP for five years was about 15 percent lower than that of similar patients not receiving CPAP. Surgical treatment of sleep apnea has a similar beneficial effect on the survival rate of patients with sleep apnea.

In France, Dr. Jean Krieger and colleagues studied 547 patients who were interviewed before treatment and at three, six, and twelve months after treatment. They not only found that treatment with CPAP reduced snoring and apnea, but also that 87 percent of the people who used CPAP had more energy and less daytime sleepiness and fatigue. Another impressive result, which they reported at the 1997 annual meeting of the Association of Professional Sleep Societies in San Francisco, was a striking reduction in accidents at home, on the road, and at work during the year in treatment. Patients had a whopping 675 near miss accidents and 94 real accidents due to impaired vigilance before treatment, but only 58 near miss and 40 real accidents during the year in treatment. Similar results were found in other studies.

To date there have been many studies showing that sleep apnea patients treated with CPAP benefit greatly from this treatment. Even after only a few nights with CPAP, many patients will feel much more alert and energetic during the day and less tired and sleepy than before the initiation of treatment. Ability to concentrate and attention span are improved. Even interest in sex may increase and sexual performance may become better.

People with sleep apnea and other medical problems may also notice improvement in their other symptoms after being treated with CPAP. For example, those with acid regurgitation, called *gastroesophageal reflux,* may note reduction in their heartburn. Those with heart problems may note so much improvement in their heart function that they can reduce or even discontinue some of their heart medications. If you are depressed and have sleep apnea, treatment of sleep apnea is likely to improve or may even completely eliminate your depression.

In 1997 a study was made of patients at a headache clinic who for a long time had had headaches during the night or upon arising in the morning. More than half of them unknowingly had sleep disorders, including many with apnea and a sleep disorder called "periodic leg movement," in which the arms or legs move restlessly throughout the night, disturbing the person's sleep. The headache patients found to have sleep apnea (many of whom had been wrongly given sleeping pills before coming to the clinic and two of whom had become addicted to painkillers because of no improvement) were treated with CPAP. In *all of them* there was complete disappearance of headache.

Another study, at the Royal Prince Alfred Hospital and Institute of Respiratory Medicine in Sydney, Australia, similarly found improvement of asthma after CPAP treatment for sleep apnea. Patients studied had both apnea and asthma, and all of the patients had heavy snoring, nighttime choking, and frequent nighttime asthma attacks, which sometimes required being rushed to the hospital. (Asthma is typically worse at night.) It turned out not only that it was safe to use the CPAP in asthma patients, but that the asthma attacks decreased in the night, and surprisingly also in the day.

CPAP can also help with nightmares. Doctors at the Minneapolis Veterans Affairs Medical Center and the University of Minnesota Medical School did studies on CPAP treatment in former prisoners of war from World War II and the Korean War who still had posttraumatic stress disorder with frequent nightmares. One 70-year-old man had been in captivity for seven months following six months of combat in Europe, a 75-year-old man had been held in captivity for forty months in the Philippine Islands and Japan following five months of combat, and a 75-year-old man had been in captivity for forty-one months in the Philippine Islands and Japan after five months of combat. When the men were treated with CPAP for their apnea, they had significantly better sleep and fewer nightmares.

But in order to derive these benefits, you usually must wear the CPAP equipment nightly. The machine does you no good staying in the closet. If you are using CPAP, remind yourself of the benefits of CPAP and have regular follow-up at your sleep clinic to help you with compliance.

If you use a CPAP, you may want to join the American Sleep Apnea Association to get their *Wellness Letter for Snoring and Apnea* so that you can keep up with the latest advice and research developments. They also have a network of support groups in many areas.

Oral Appliances

We told you in the previous chapter about some of the early medical appliances to help stop snoring: facial masks, chin straps, and bandages that wrapped around the head and held up the lower jaw. Most of them used mouthpieces or other devices to apply pressure on the chin to keep the mouth closed, or to train the sleeper to breathe through the nose.

Things are different now.

Today there are several dozen modern oral appliances designed to keep the mouth shut, to move the jaw forward, or to prevent the tongue from falling backward. They are designed to help stop mouth breathing, reduce the crowding of the airway, and allow air to flow more freely. These modern-day appliances include the Herbst appliance, the tongue positioner and exerciser, the Hilsen adjustable positioner, the Thornton adjustable positioner, the Klearway appliance, the Jasper jumper, the Esmarch appliance, and many more. Some of the appliance names are a bit scary—the Equalizer, the Silencer—but despite their names, they are often helpful for both snoring and apnea.

The American Sleep Disorders Association (ASDA) in 1995 released a report on standards of practice for various oral appliances. The ASDA investigators reviewed twenty-one publications of research reports on oral appliances and reported that in nearly all who used an oral appliance, it reduced or eradicated their snoring, and in most cases, the appliances also reduced the frequency of episodes of apnea (but up to 40 percent still had some apnea or partial apnea).

Based on these studies, the ASDA currently recommends that oral appliances are appropriate for

> patients who snore or who have mild obstructive sleep apnea and for whom weight loss or changing their sleep position has not worked,
>
> patients with moderate to severe sleep apnea who refuse or cannot use CPAP, and
>
> patients who refuse or are not logical candidates for surgery.

How to Use an Oral Appliance

Once an oral appliance has been chosen as the method of therapy, the ASDA recommends that it be fitted by a qualified person, usually a dentist who has had appropriate training.

There are considerable differences in the design of oral appliances and how they work in different patients. Your dentist will need to examine your mouth and teeth to determine which appliance is best for you. The goal of the appliances is to modify the position of the tongue and jaw so as to enlarge the airway or make it less collapsible.

For all appliances, proper fitting and alignment is important, so be sure to have your work done by someone experienced in the field. It may take several visits and adjustments to get your appliance to fit comfortably; the less bulky, the better. A nonporous material is best for easy cleaning and protection against germs and odor. And you need to have instruction in proper use. Also keep in mind that for a few patients, the appliances make snoring and apnea worse, so after you have the appliance fitted it is important to have regular checkups and report back to your doctor whether your symptoms have improved, or have returned, become worse, or changed in any way. Because snoring and apnea have medical implications, the dentist providing treatment should always be in close communication with your physician.

Some patients are only able to use the appliances for a few hours at night at first, but later, as they become used to them, they can wear them the entire night.

Oral appliances of various kinds have been effective in reducing or eliminating snoring in most patients (50 percent of patients in some studies, 75 percent in another, 100 percent in another). Often they are also effective against apnea, reducing episodes on average to half of what they were before the appliance; however, in some patients apnea stayed the same or became worse. Most, but not all, patients have reported a reduction of daytime sleepiness.

Possible side effects include sore teeth and gums, pain in the jaw joint, and excessive salivation (drooling). The ASDA says that oral appliances may aggravate temporomandibular joint (TMJ) disease and may cause dental misalignment and discomfort in patients with TMJ. Follow-up care by a dentist is essential to watch for any complications.

Costs can range from $50 to $2,000, depending on the quality of materials and how much custom fitting needs to be done. The cheaper devices should not be used if you have extensive dental work or problems, such as bridges or missing teeth, but you need to be careful of dental work with even the most expensive devices. Talk to your dentist about potential damage in your present dental situation.

Types of Devices

There are two major types of oral appliances: those that act on the tongue and those that act on the jaw.

Tongue-Retaining Devices

Tongue-retaining devices (TRDs) were the first oral appliances to be developed and used. They work by keeping the tongue forward.

In 1982 Drs. Rosalind Cartwright and Herbert Samelson in Chicago devised a TRD designed to keep the tongue from falling backward and narrowing the airway, thus allowing better airflow. This device keeps the tongue from falling back in the throat by means of negative pressure in a soft plastic air bubble, held in place in front of the teeth by a flange that fits between the lips and teeth. The patient sucks the air out of the bubble, inserts the tongue, and the negative pressure in the bubble holds the tongue forward for several hours.

The TRD devised by Drs. Cartwright and Samelson was effective in reducing the number of episodes of complete or incomplete stopped breathing to about half of what they were before using the device.

Other TRDs have been developed and tested in a few apnea patients. For example, in 1987 Dr. Peter George of the University of Hawaii described a nocturnal airway patency appliance (NAPA) made of wire and acrylic that keeps the airway open during sleep by pushing the tongue forward. It also moves the lower jaw forward, although less so than mandibular advancement devices. In one study of sixteen patients the NAPA appliance reduced the number of stopped-breathing episodes from thirty-seven per hour to nine per hour. Not all TRDs are effective; for example, another device, called SnorEx, manufactured in Germany, failed to improve the number of stopped-breathing episodes in the majority of patients tested.

Overall, only in less than half of patients do TRDs reduce the number of stopped-breathing episodes to less than ten per hour of sleep, which is considered normal. Long-term compliance with these devices has not yet been assessed systematically. There are individual patients who have used them for many years, but the overall acceptance rate appears to be no better than 50 percent. They work best in patients whose snoring is worse when sleeping on the back.

Many patients complain about tongue discomfort when using TRDs. Even when these devices work effectively, many patients do not continue to use them. Too many patients have found them uncomfortable. According to a recent survey conducted by Dr. Daniel Loube of the Walter Reed Army Medical Center in Washington, D.C., tongue-retaining devices make up 7 percent of the dental appliances used today.

Mandibular Advancement Appliances

Mandibular advancement appliances (MAAs), sometimes called mandibular advancement splints or jaw retainers, are the most common devices used today. They have been studied—and used—much more extensively than tongue-retaining devices, and the results with using them are better than with TRDs. MAAs usually consist of two dental plates made by taking a dental impression of the upper and lower teeth. They are made of acrylic materials, which are molded to conform to the patient's teeth and the shape of the mouth. They usually have some retention clasps to keep them in place. When the device is inserted into the mouth, the lower plate pushes the lower jaw forward, which also makes the tongue protrude, thus preventing airway narrowing during sleep. Some MAAs allow for adjustment of the position for the lower jaw, thus permitting adjustment to the individual patient and minimizing discomfort. Most devices need to be custom-fitted, requiring molding and manufacturing in a dental laboratory, although there are now some devices available in prefabricated form that can be molded to the patient's teeth in the dentist's office. When first worn, MAAs usually feel uncomfortable and require adjustment by the dentist. On average, about three visits to the dentist are necessary to achieve proper fit. MAAs only need to be worn at night, but some patients initially also wear them for an hour or two during the day, simply to get used to them.

The first MAA was described by Dr. K. Meier-Ewart in Germany, and was used in 1986 by Dr. W. Kloss in a study of seven patients with sleep apnea. In the next year Dr. Meier-Ewart studied the same appliance in forty-four patients. Over the next ten years, many more studies were done using different types of MAA. Of three hundred patients now studied overall, in more than half their stopped-breathing episodes were reduced to the normal range—less than ten per hour. Most important, the patients tolerated these appliances much better than the tongue-retaining devices. In fact, 77 percent of patients were continuing to use their appliances at the two-year follow-up. Because of the small number of patients studied in each series, it is not possible to state with any confidence which is the best appliance.

Comparing tongue-retaining devices with mandibular advancement appliances, it is seen that MAAs do a better job of eliminating snoring and decreasing the number of stopped-breathing episodes, they get the most patients to what is considered a normal level of episodes, and they have a higher patient acceptance rate.

Some MAAs have clasps and elastic bands that restrict mouth opening, while others allow relatively unhindered mouth opening. Some designs include tubes or openings for breathing. Some also have an extension toward the back that is designed to modify the position of the soft palate or tongue.

All of the early MAA appliances were of a fixed type; that is, the only way to change the relative position of the jaw was to remold the entire appliance. But in 1990 Dr. Allan Lowe, a dentist at the University of

British Columbia in Vancouver, developed an adjustable mandibular advancement appliance. It is called the Klearway appliance to emphasize that it can keep the airway clear and unobstructed. The Klearway appliance allows the dentist to adjust the position of the lower jaw by moving the appliance forward or backward a few millimeters to ensure the most comfort or to improve the MAA's effectiveness. However, once the appliance is in the mouth, if you feel uncomfortable and need to adjust the lower jaw position, the appliance has to be taken out of the mouth because the adjustment is made from the back. That is why Dr. Keith Thornton of Dallas, Texas, developed another adjustable appliance, called the Thornton Adjustable Positioner (TAP), in which the adjustment can be done from the front of the mouth using a screw that is part of the appliance. Initial adjustments to the appliance are done by the dentist. Later, fine-tuning can be done by the patient by simply turning the screw a few turns to move the lower plate forward or backward. Another new adjustable jaw positioner, called the Silencer, was developed by Dr. Wayne Halstrom of Vancouver, British Columbia. The Silencer has a unique titanium hinge that allows the lower jaw to advance over a range of 10 mm (0.39 inch).

Effects of Oral Appliances

No matter what oral appliance is used, they all seem to improve and often eliminate snoring and improve apnea in most patients. They are definitely a useful alternative for those patients with sleep apnea who cannot tolerate CPAP therapy, and they are the treatment of choice for snorers without sleep apnea if they still require treatment after carrying out the weight loss and other lifestyle changes recommended.

One study of a fixed-type mandibular appliance, called Snor-Guard, that was used by sixty-eight men and women who suffered from loud snoring and varying degrees of sleep apnea found that snoring was eliminated in 42 percent of the patients and was decreased in the rest. Choking, apnea, awakenings, and daytime sleepiness were also eliminated in many of the patients. The symptoms returned on the nights when the device was not used. Side effects included mouth discomfort and excessive salivation, but at follow-up several months later, three out of four patients were still using the appliance.

Another study was made of sixty-one patients who had problems with snoring and obstructive sleep apnea that was not serious enough for them to use CPAP, or who had refused to use CPAP or could not tolerate it. (Three of the patients were unable to tolerate the appliance because they had no teeth.) Snoring improved with the oral appliance in all cases where the bedpartner could be interviewed. Two out of three patients reported jaw discomfort, but this disappeared in many of the patients after three weeks, and 79 percent of the patients continued to use the device regularly. There was also significant improvement in the patients' apnea.

A dentist colleague in Toronto, Dr. Jeffrey Pancer, worked with Dr. Hoffstein at St. Michael's Hospital in studying a group of thirty-four patients with snoring and sleep apnea. They found that when an adjustable-type oral appliance was used, stopped breathing was reduced from forty-two episodes per hour to eleven per hour on average. And the appliance did not interfere with sleep. In the sleep laboratory, patients fell asleep within nineteen minutes of turning off the lights, slept for about six hours, did not have an unduly large number of awakenings after falling asleep, and were able to achieve stages of deep sleep. After they had worn the appliances at night for more than two months, the patients were asked about side effects or discomfort. Out of the thirty-eight patients, ten reported frequent teeth discomfort or a feeling that their teeth were apart, and about one out of four reported excessive salivation or jaw pain. Only a few reported occasional gum or tongue discomfort. Before the appliance was applied and two months later, bedpartners were asked whether they were disturbed by snoring. Before the appliance was used, 93 percent of the bedpartners said the patient often snored loudly, frequently keeping them awake and sometimes forcing them to sleep in another room. With the appliance, the bedpartners said snoring occurred sometimes, rarely, or not at all. When patients were asked whether they were satisfied with the oral appliance, almost 90 percent were either very or moderately satisfied, and only a few patients were dissatisfied.

Excessive salivation often occurs in the beginning of using an MAA, but usually disappears after a brief time. Occasionally, but not usually, there may be jaw pain or changes in bite alignment.

As for tongue-retaining devices, they are for most people not as effective as the mandibular advancement appliances.

There are other oral appliances besides tongue-retaining devices and mandibular advancement appliances—for example, lip shields, appliances that extend the palate, and palate lifters—but none of these have been tested extensively.

Recommendations

Where does all this take us in the treatment spectrum of patients with snoring or sleep apnea?

The first thing to do if you have snoring *without apnea* is to follow the recommendations for changes in your lifestyle, as we outlined in the first few chapters. Don't drink or take sleeping pills or tranquilizers to help you sleep; stop smoking; and very important, lose weight. Also check for allergies or other things possibly causing nasal obstruction, don't sleep on your back, and breathe with your mouth closed.

If these changes have not worked, you can try the nasal dilators and other simple aids we talked about in the previous chapter. And if all these things have not stopped your snoring, the next step is to talk with a sleep specialist about using an oral appliance. Of the oral appliances, mandibular advancement appliances, whether fixed or adjustable, are usually the most effective and are the most commonly used ones today. Tongue-retaining devices are a secondary choice. However, you should go to a dentist who has experience with oral appliances. The dentist will examine your mouth and teeth and can better decide which appliance, if any, is best for you.

The next thing to try is a continuous positive airway pressure (CPAP) machine. If it doesn't work, you can consider surgery.

If you have snoring *with apnea,* particularly if apnea is severe, then you need to make the same lifestyle modifications as in snoring without apnea—don't use alcohol or sleeping pills before bed; don't smoke; lose weight. And as in snoring without apnea, check for allergies. The next recommended step is to try CPAP. If you are not able to tolerate that, the alternative is to try one of the oral appliances. If neither CPAP nor oral appliances work for you, then surgery should be considered. But remember that before giving up on CPAP, you must make sure that you had an optimum trial of it; that is, you had the proper mask and headgear, a humidifier, ramping, and the pressure on the blower was not too low or too high.

If you think you might need help from an oral appliance or a CPAP device, be sure to check with your physician, dentist, or a sleep specialist first. You need to be referred to a professional who is knowledgeable about CPAP and oral appliances and who has had plenty of experience in working with them and in dealing with the various problems and concerns that can arise at follow-up. It is possible that using the newest materials and paying careful attention to customized fitting of the devices will reduce the side effects and improve compliance.

It is necessary to have individual attention, and often the devices need to be modified. The effectiveness of one device over another, whether CPAP or oral appliance, will vary among individual patients, depending on their particular anatomical features.

Much research still needs to be done, especially in long-term follow-up and in comparing the success rates of various devices and of the devices versus surgery. (We will tell you about the latest surgical methods in the final chapter.)

10

If You Go
to a Sleep Lab

We hope that by following the lifestyle changes and other simple steps in our program, you have overcome your snoring. Most people on the program have success without ever going to a sleep lab or sleep disorders center.

A few people, however, do need to go. Fortunately, there are now many labs and centers throughout the world, and more than three hundred in the United States (see Appendix A). Here are the situations in which you should talk to your doctor about going to a sleep lab for further investigation:

- If your snoring is serious, and you have not been able to solve the problem by losing weight, stopping cigarettes, and stopping nighttime drinking, sleeping pills, and tranquilizers
- If you have frequent or long-lasting stopped-breathing episodes
- If you have great difficulty staying awake during the day, especially if you are so excessively sleepy in the daytime that you are in danger of an accident at work, at home, or on the road
- If you experience marked mental difficulties such as forgetfulness or disorientation along with your sleep problem
- If your snoring has jeopardized a job or a social relationship
- If you feel or someone has said that there is something seriously abnormal about your sleep, such as breathing difficulties or leg twitching

If any of these problems exist, you should discuss it with your doctor for a referral to a sleep disorders center where your condition can be investigated further.

If You Go to a Sleep Disorders Center

Once you've decided to go to a center, how do you get in? It's usually best to get a referral from your physician. That way, the center won't need to repeat tests that have already been done by your doctor and can refer its findings back to your doctor. However, some centers will make appointments directly with patients.

Appendix A provides the official list of centers accredited by the American Sleep Disorders Association (ASDA). This means that these centers have been checked by the ASDA as meeting high standards. Every month, new centers are added, so write to the ASDA if no center is listed for your area. Their address is in Appendix B (or check their web site at www.asda.org). Appendix B also provides a list of sources to contact for names of centers in other countries.

The following description, adapted from *No More Sleepless Nights* by Dr. Peter Hauri, head of the Sleep Disorders Center of the Mayo Clinic in Rochester, Minnesota, and Dr. Linde, will give you an accurate idea of what to expect at a center.

Most sleep disorders centers look pretty much alike and do about the same things. Usually, you'll be sent a Sleep Log and a Sleep Questionnaire. Once you've filled out the questionnaire and kept the log for a week or two, and your doctor has sent the center a summary of your medical record, the center will set up an interview.

At the interview, a sleep specialist will ask you questions to find out more about how you sleep, psychological and social issues, and your ideas and feelings about your sleep problem. It's important to be forthright with the sleep specialist. Small details can be important, and no matter how unusual or personal you think something is, your sleep specialist probably has heard it before. If you leave something out, that one fact could be the key to evaluating your problem.

After the interview, which may last fifteen to ninety minutes, the specialist will decide whether you need to sleep overnight in the lab. If you do sleep in the lab, you might be asked to stay the following day to complete a multiple sleep latency test (MSLT). This is the test that measures how sleepy you are during the day by having you go to bed at two-hour intervals and seeing whether and how fast you fall asleep.

Finally, you may have a follow-up visit with the sleep specialist to discuss the center's findings and recommendations for your sleep problem. Or, if you were referred by a physician, the center might simply report this information to your physician.

Sleeping in the Lab

Many people ask, "How can I ever sleep in the lab with wires attached to me and somebody watching me, when I can't even sleep at home?"

In our experience, this is almost never a problem. In fact, many insomniacs sleep much better in the lab than at home, and it's hard to find what's wrong with their sleep when they sleep so well. Even if you turn out to be the rare person who does have trouble sleeping in the lab, it's okay—you're there so they can find out about your bad sleep. You'll be giving them plenty to measure and study.

Coming to the Lab

You should not take any naps during the day before coming to the lab. Unless otherwise instructed, do not use alcohol, stimulants, or sedatives twenty-four hours before the study, including not drinking any coffee or tea in the afternoon or evening. If you're using sleeping pills every night, check with the lab if you should take them that night. (Many labs require that you stop taking all sleeping pills for two to three weeks before the lab study.) Check with the sleep disorders center regarding what to do about other medications you take regularly. You may eat a normal evening meal before coming in. Bring comfortable sleep attire (with robe and socks or slippers for walking around in the halls or sitting in the TV room if there is one) and personal hygiene items you need at bedtime and in the morning. When you get to your room, you will be asked to fill out a presleep questionnaire that asks what you have done during the day and whether you have taken any medication that day or recently.

What the Sleep Technician Does

After you get into your pajamas and are ready for bed, a sleep technician will attach various electrodes. These are little metal cups, smaller than a dime, filled with jelly and attached to very flexible wires. The first ones are attached to your head and measure your brain waves both while you are awake and during your various sleep stages. This recording is called an electroencephalogram, or EEG. Depending on the lab, anywhere from two to six electrodes may be glued to your scalp with collodion or some other substance. (The collodion is removed the next morning with acetone; if any remains, you can use nail polish remover at home to get it out.)

An oxymeter may be attached to your finger or earlobe to measure how well your blood is saturated with oxygen. When blood carries more oxygen, it is redder, and when blood carries less oxygen, it is bluer. Some oxymeters do not use a visible light, but the principle is the same: the oxymeter determines how well your blood is oxygenated during sleep. If you have apnea, this often helps to determine how serious the apnea might be.

There will be other electrodes alongside your eyes to measure your eye movements (electrooculogram, or EOG). Electrodes on your chin will measure muscle tension and relaxation (electromyogram, or EMG). The EMG is especially important during REM sleep to see whether your muscles are paralyzed, as they should be in REM sleep. (REM stands for rapid eye movement.)

Sensors are placed in front of your nostrils and mouth to measure the temperature just outside your nose and mouth, which reflects airflow. (The temperature is cooler when you inhale and warmer when you exhale, and from this we can tell whether air is actually moving through your nostrils and mouth.) Two bands are usually applied to measure breathing movement, one around your abdomen and one around your chest. With these bands, we can get a feeling for how much air is actually being moved, or whether you are trying to breathe but cannot because you have sleep apnea caused by some obstruction. (Some labs measure the same thing with electrodes applied to the skin between the ribs, where they measure muscle contractions and relaxations when you try to breathe.)

Electrodes are applied to your legs to measure whether your legs twitch during sleep. Finally, electrodes are placed on your chest or back to record your heart rate and rhythm.

All these measurements are more or less standard for any patient in any lab. But sometimes there are additions and variations. For example, if there is a chance that you might be having seizures at night, you will have extra electrodes applied to your scalp to make additional measurements of brain waves. In some cases where a diagnosis is difficult, a small catheter might be inserted through your nose and fairly far down your throat to measure the pressure there and assess breathing effort. That is done relatively rarely, however, and it is much less uncomfortable than it sounds. In some labs there may be a microphone to measure snoring sounds.

You will sleep in a regular bed in a private bedroom, and there will be a place to hang your clothes. The wires will be plugged into special outlets at the head of your bed, and feed into various recording instruments in the monitoring room. This room looks like a miniature version of Mission Control, with recording instruments busily tracing the physiology of each sleeping patient. Technicians monitor the recordings from this room. They keep an all-night vigil, charting the brain wave activity as each sleeper passes through the various stages of sleep. Then they calculate various measurements for the sleep specialists to study the next morning.

(You might want to know that in an accredited sleep lab, the technicians who work with you are well trained. There is now an Association of Polysomnographic Technologists that gives exams, and many of the technicians who work with you have been certified by that organization. They know what they are doing, and you are in safe hands in the lab—probably safer there than if you were sleeping at home, because somebody is always awake in the lab making sure everything is okay.)

Don't worry that you might receive a shock from any of the wires attached to you. The instruments are set up to measure the electricity you produce—they don't put out any electricity that could shock you.

Once the electrodes and sensors are connected, the technician flips a switch, and the recording begins. Formerly the recordings were made with at least eight pens scratching back and forth on a moving stack of paper, making long, scribbly lines of waves and peaks and squiggles.

Today, most labs use computers. In the noncomputerized method, the recordings are linked across a long, continuous paper about 2 feet wide and 1,000 feet long. In the computerized method, the same amount of information moves across the computer screen. The computer has the advantage of being able to automatically analyze many of the events in the record, and recording speeds can be changed to look at important events in different ways. Moreover, a computer does not use up all the paper that is needed by the old method.

You and the technician will talk back and forth on the microphone in your room for a few minutes to test the quality of the recordings. The technician usually checks while your eyes are open and closed, while moving your eyes to the right and left, while breathing, while holding your breath, while tensing and relaxing your leg muscles, and so on.

In your bed, you can move around easily and twist and turn as much as you want—the electrodes are attached to very flexible wires. You do have to get unplugged to go to the bathroom, because the wires are not that long. But don't worry, in all sleep disorders centers there is a technician on duty all night monitoring the equipment, and your room microphone will be turned on all night. If you want to get up, you simply call, and the technician comes and unplugs the wires so you can go to the bathroom. Don't worry about how often you need to call for assistance. Some patients are so nervous that they have to go to the bathroom ten to fifteen times, and it's the technician's job to unplug you however many times you need to get up.

Some laboratories have setups for video recording, so there might be an infrared light and a video camera in your room. That is because the technicians need to know what positions you lie in during the night. Some people snore only on their backs, and some people twitch violently while sleeping. Some labs also have specially designed position monitors that record what position you're lying in.

The Record

If you were to look at a recording of your sleep stages, you would see that the brain waves on the EEG at first are fast and small, indicating that you are awake. When you get drowsy, regular and larger waves appear, about ten per second. In the transition between sleeping and waking, the waves become slower, about three to seven per second. As you fall asleep, the recording of the eye movements (EOG) shows slow rolls as the eyes move back and forth. The first signs on the EEG that you are actually asleep are the sleep spindles, displaying quick bursts of rapid waves, like crescendos and decrescendos in a musical performance.

Soon, the record shows bursts of spindle waves interspersed with larger, slower waves, occurring at about one per second. As these large waves, called *delta waves,* become more frequent, you rarely move. You are in a deep delta sleep. This is the best sleep of the night, when most bodily recovery occurs. You may spend five to ninety minutes in delta sleep.

About ninety minutes after you fall asleep, you enter a new stage. Your brain waves begin to look as if you are almost awake. Your eyes move under your closed lids, as if you're looking around. You are dreaming and your muscles are paralyzed to prevent you from carrying out your dreams. This is REM sleep.

As the night goes on, you have less and less delta sleep, and a dream occurs about every ninety minutes. The first one lasts only about five minutes and usually is boring, a rehash of something you did that day. Every dream gets a little longer and more exciting than the previous one. If you sleep six hours a night, you probably have four dreams.

Another thing we see on the EEG is that everybody, even the best sleeper, wakes up three to eight times each hour. Typically, a good sleeper comes just barely to consciousness for two to four seconds and then falls asleep again, never to remember the awakening. However, if something untoward is perceived—for example, a sound or smell that should not be there, or a sensation that the bed is too hot or too cold— then you wake up fully so you can do something about it. These three to eight short awakenings per hour in normal sleepers are simply for safety. However, the poor sleeper, on some of these awakenings, imme- diately snaps to full attention, looks at the clock, or worries why he is awake again, and then often has problems getting back to sleep.

Things are not quiet in the land of Morpheus. The average sleeper hardly betrays the busy brain activity going on within. But in the sleep labs, EEG recordings clearly document this activity. As one sleep re- searcher said, "It's not like parking your brain in the garage for the night. Things are going on!"

The EEG brain wave charts represent the brain's computing appa- ratus at work. The brain, which looks like a head of a cauliflower, and is gray and squishy to the touch, contains over 15 billion nerve cells, with long fibers of nerve cells linking to other nerve cells in an interweaving jungle of switchboard connections. Messages of sights, sounds, smells, happiness, and pain flash through the connections at breathtaking speed. And in billions of cells are stored memories, emotions, facts, be- liefs, reasoning—all the factors that help shape our personalities. Also among those brain cells are the centers that control body functions such as breathing, heartbeat, vision, and speech—as well as waking and sleeping. It's an impressive computer you spend the night with.

The Analysis

In the morning, your electrodes are removed. You then fill out a questionnaire in which you are asked how you felt about the night, how long you thought it took to fall asleep, how many hours you thought you slept, and so on. This is to compare what you felt was happening with what the recordings actually show. In some cases, what patients believe happened is different from what actually happened. It is important to know the actual facts, for example, whether you slept four hours but feel that you slept seven hours, or slept four hours but feel you didn't sleep at all.

In the morning, sleep specialists scrutinize the recording that was made all night and study the summaries and charts that the technicians have put together. They see how long it took you to fall asleep, how long you spent in the different stages of sleep, when you were dreaming and when you were not, whether you snored, whether your legs or arms twitched, what your breathing was like, whether you had stopped-breathing episodes and how often and whether breathing was correlated with times you woke up. You then have a meeting about the findings and talk about possible treatments.

11

Surgical
Treatments

For many, surgery is the cure for their snoring problems.

This was true of Kent, a retired executive with a fifty-foot sailboat, who had much to offer including an excellent disposition, a sense of adventure, and dancing skills. But he kept any serious life partners away because they were blasted sleepless when his stentorian snores sounded throughout the staterooms of his boat. Kent tried everything, including losing weight, but the snoring persisted. He went for medical consultation. Together, he and the doctor decided surgery might be the answer in his set of circumstances. He had the surgery and it changed his life.

Surgery as a treatment for snoring has received a great deal of attention during the last two decades. And its use has increased as the public has become more aware that snoring can lead to apnea and other adverse health consequences, and as frustrated bedpartners have decided they can no longer put up with sleepless nights. Now snorers and their bedpartners are beginning to talk to their family doctors about the snoring problems disrupting their lives and what can be done.

Given the rather limited choice of treatment options and the difficulties in complying with the lifestyle modifications that help, such as weight loss and cessation of alcohol and sleeping pills, surgery seems to offer simple, quick, and permanent relief.

However, as experience with surgery grows, it becomes apparent that surgery is not an option that is best for every snorer. There are some snorers who are better candidates for surgery than others. In this chapter we will describe the various types of surgery and the latest information that is known about each.

Nose Surgery

If you have an obvious anatomical deformity in your nasal passages that causes narrowing, thus setting up conditions favorable for vibrations lower down, you have a better chance of benefiting from surgery than those who do not have any obvious anatomical deformities. Deformities of the nose are some of the most easily recognized and treated, and surgery to correct those abnormalities can have excellent results.

For example, snorers may have narrowing of the nasal passages due to a deviated septum, a broken nose, nasal polyps, or enlarged adenoids. If one of these is the reason for your snoring, you have a good chance of either getting rid of your snoring completely or greatly improving it by surgical correction of the anatomical problem. A deviated septum can be straightened, a broken nose fixed, polyps treated, and enlarged adenoids removed.

All of these procedures are usually done by an ear, nose, and throat (ENT) specialist in a hospital setting. The surgery is almost always done from underneath or inside the nose, leaving no visible scars. Either local or general anesthesia can be used.

Both personal stories and scientific studies have shown that there are good results in curing snoring when nasal abnormalities are corrected. One of the better-known scientific reports is that of Dr. David Fairbanks of George Washington University School of Medicine in Washington, D.C. Dr. Fairbanks performed nasal surgery in forty-seven snorers (twenty-nine of whom snored occasionally, eighteen constantly); about one year later these patients were asked about their snoring, and thirty-six of them said that their snoring was either eliminated or improved—a 77 percent success rate. In another well-known study, Dr. C. Woodhead at Leeds General Infirmary in the United Kingdom operated on twenty-nine snorers and found improvement or resolution of snoring in twenty—a 69 percent success rate.

It is not known to what extent snoring recurs several years after nasal surgery, because there have been no really long-term follow-up studies. But at St. Michael's, our general impression is that initially after surgery snoring improves markedly during the first six to twelve months in at least 80 percent of patients, but later it recurs in many of them. Sometimes the reason is weight gain, alcohol, or recurrence of polyps, but sometimes there is not an obvious reason. Overall, it is our impression that nasal surgery, even if performed in properly selected candidates, has at best a 50 percent success rate in curing snoring over the long term, mostly because the patients allow themselves to gain weight or fall back into other unhealthy snore-producing habits.

If you have nasal obstruction and you snore, it is a good idea to go to a specialist to have this checked, even if you are afraid or apprehensive about surgery. Indeed, you may find that your fears are unnecessary—not all cases of nasal obstruction require surgery, and many can be treated medically. The doctor may tell you that your nose is stuffy because the lining is inflamed due to allergies, postnasal drip, or even for no obvious reason. The problem can often be solved by treatment with nasal sprays—decongestants or steroids—often within days.

Or it may be obvious that surgery is the best chance of eliminating your snoring. Your physician will refer you to a specialist in your area who is best qualified to evaluate your case and do the surgery. Or if swollen tissue inside the nose is the cause, the tissue can sometimes be shrunk by simple laser treatment done in the physician's office or by cryosurgery, a procedure that takes less than thirty minutes.

Sometimes there can be deformities of the nose that are not so obvious. These defects can cause unrealized narrowing of the airway. Some of the newer techniques of CAT scans and radiography can now find these hidden defects so that they can be corrected.

Enlarged Tonsils and Adenoids

People who have enlarged tonsils or adenoids will also usually benefit from surgery. Enlarged tonsils and adenoids are frequently the cause of snoring and apnea in children. And in most cases, removing the enlarged tonsils and adenoids will promptly cure children's snoring and apnea.

Children generally should not have tonsillectomy or adenoidectomy before the age of 3. The operation, called "T and A" by surgeons when done together, is one of the most frequent procedures performed in children. In general, if the tonsils are removed, the adenoids are removed also. Obstructed breathing during sleep is one of the major indications for the surgery. The procedure is done in the hospital, often on an outpatient basis or with a one-night stay for observation. It usually takes six to eight weeks after surgery for snoring and apnea symptoms to disappear.

If your child frequently snores at night, suffers from headaches, usually breathes through his mouth instead of his nose, is restless at night, and wakes up with a dry mouth, you should have him examined by a physician for the possibility of enlarged tonsils and adenoids or some other anatomical problem that impedes proper breathing. Amazingly, this set of warning signs was first described in 1858 by a German physician, Dr. Friedrich Betz, but it is still sometimes not recognized as a problem by parents whose children snore. It is important for parents to recognize snoring and apnea problems and seek appropriate help for their children.

It is not normal for a child to snore loudly and constantly. If your child snores, do not hesitate in obtaining medical advice. Give your child love and understanding since he cannot control the condition, and seek proper treatment for him. When you take your child in for a regular medical checkup, even if not asked, be sure to tell the doctor about snoring, gasping for breath, apnea, or even restlessness and strange sleeping positions.

In addition to snoring, 1 to 3 percent of children also have apnea. It can occur in any child from newborn to teenager, but is most prevalent at 2 to 6 years of age. This too is usually due to large tonsils and adenoids. However, some children with huge tonsils do not have snoring or apnea, while some with small tonsils and adenoids do. There is no set pattern.

T and A should not be done routinely, but when there is severe snoring and apnea, the procedure will cure it in most children.

A sidelight: children who snore are often bed wetters. In fact, bedwetting in young adults is a strong indicator of sleep apnea. Almost always, after a T and A, sleep quality improves and bedwetting typically disappears.

In addition, since many children who snore or have apnea also have daytime fatigue and sleepiness, this is often cured after a T and A. One wonders how many of the children who are thought to be lazy, unmotivated, or stupid are really suffering from excessive daytime sleepiness because they are not sleeping through the night. A study at the University of Michigan has also implicated apnea as a possible factor in some cases of hyperactivity in children. If your child is having trouble at school, listen to him breathe at night. Curing his apnea might change his life.

Early Surgery

Early in the history of surgery for snoring, surgical procedures to cure snoring concentrated on the removal of the uvula, the piece of tissue that hangs down in the back of the throat. Most people who snore do not have an obvious anatomical abnormality, but they usually have a very bulky, swollen, and inflamed uvula. If you are like many people who are heavy snorers or who have apnea, you can look into a mirror and see just how swollen and enlarged your uvula looks as it hangs down from the roof of your mouth. You can easily imagine how it can block the airway and vibrate during sleep to cause snoring and apnea.

One of the first ENT surgeons who started operating on the throat almost forty years ago to cure snoring was Dr. Takenosuke Ikematsu of Japan. He examined many adult snorers and was impressed by the fact that more than 90 percent of them appeared to have a narrow throat, with a long uvula and a thick soft palate (the soft part of the roof of the mouth). He removed the uvula and part of the soft palate and found that in many patients snoring was cured. Dr. Ikematsu published his results in 1964, reporting that in 152 snorers operated on, 82 percent had relief from their snoring. At the time of his studies there was as yet no awareness of sleep apnea.

But as others tried the operation, not everybody agreed with Dr. Ikematsu's conclusions, and some physicians said that most of the operations on the uvula and soft palate seemed irrational or unjustified and rarely gave relief.

A few years later, when sleep apnea was discovered, there was a renewed interest in finding a cure for serious snoring and apnea. One surgical procedure devised was a tracheostomy. This operation creates a hole in the windpipe, just below the level of the Adam's apple. The hole is plugged up with a special stopper during the day, and is opened at night for sleeping. The person can breathe through the hole while sleeping, bypassing any obstruction or narrowing above this level that might be interfering with breathing. This operation always cures snoring and apnea, but clearly it is not something that most of us would eagerly accept. Aside from serious aesthetic problems, there can be serious medical complications, such as infection at the place where the hole is made, which can spread to other parts of the windpipe; scarring of the tissues around the hole, which can result in a need for additional surgery; and irritation of tissue by the air being breathed directly into the windpipe without being warmed up and humidified as it would if it passed through the nose and throat. And the patient could be in danger of secretions plugging up the windpipe, which potentially could even be fatal.

Tracheostomy is very rarely performed today, and never for simple snoring. On rare occasion, it is used in patients with severe sleep apnea who cannot have any other treatment or who require a temporary measure to relieve their sleep apnea while they are awaiting another more permanent solution.

UPPP Surgery

In 1981 Dr. Shiro Fujita of Detroit, Michigan, modified the operation devised by Dr. Ikematsu to remove not only the uvula and part of the soft palate, but also the tonsils and other extra tissues from the back of the throat (the *pharynx*, in medical terminology). This operation received the long name *uvulopalatopharyngoplasty*, or *UPPP* for short. Despite the name, which undoubtedly turns off some patients, the operation is quite simple, has a low chance of serious complications, and is still widely performed today.

The operation is performed under general anesthesia. If present, the tonsils are removed, and the surgeon then removes tissue from the edge of the soft palate to expand the airway, but does not remove so much tissue as to interfere with speech or swallowing. A UPPP requires several days in the hospital.

Initially, an excellent success rate was reported; for example, in the original report of Dr. Fujita, all twelve patients who had UPPP reported improvement or disappearance of snoring. Subsequent investigations reported somewhat lower success rates. It was difficult to compare results because there was a great deal of variability between different studies—follow-up time was anywhere between four weeks and seven years, sleep studies to rule out sleep apnea before or after surgery were not consistently performed, and the methods of assessing snoring differed between the studies. At St. Michael's, we looked at fourteen studies, all done between 1981 and 1997, where the effect of UPPP on just snoring, not sleep apnea, was assessed. There was a total of 974 patients, 85 percent of whom were considered a surgical success and reported improvement or disappearance of snoring.

One of the more rigorous studies was done by Dr. Danielle Friberg and colleagues at the Karolinska Institute in Sweden. They studied fifty-six patients, all of whom snored but did not have sleep apnea. Almost all were given a second sleep study five years after the UPPP surgery and were asked about their snoring. Fifteen patients (27 percent) reported that they did not snore at all, and thirty-four (60 percent) reported that they snored less, for a total success rate of 87 percent.

Not all investigators have found such good success rates. For example, Drs. Barry Levin and Gary Becker of Kaiser Permanante Medical Center in Panorama City, California, found that although within one week of surgery 87 percent of patients reported disappearance or significant reduction in snoring, one year later this favorable success rate had dropped to 46 percent. However, researchers at Oxford, England, found that after long-term follow-up of one to seven years after UPPP, there was a 13 percent recurrence of snoring, but that the risk of recurrence was directly related to body weight. If you were fat, or became fat, you were more likely to have a return of snoring.

Side effects of UPPP, most of which are minor, are reported by up to 35 percent of patients. There is usually pain and some drooling for several weeks; other side effects can include throat irritation, nasal speech, and problems with swallowing. Very rarely there are more serious side effects such as bleeding, infection, regurgitation of liquids or foods into the nose when swallowing, or permanent speech defect. Some patients who have had much of the soft palate removed have a feeling of always wanting to clear the throat, similar to what one feels with postnasal drip.

It is not possible to predict with absolute certainty who will respond favorably to UPPP and who will not. However, it appears that people without apnea and without other risk factors (particularly obesity) have a better chance of success.

You should also remember that snoring may not be completely eliminated after surgery, but it may only be that your snoring's loudness will be reduced and its pitch changed—and this might make it more acceptable for your bedpartner.

There are several variations to the UPPP procedure, with different surgeons using different approaches and modifications of technique but the results from the different variations are too few to draw definite conclusions as to which surgical variation, if any, is superior.

There are also differences in what is done based on which parts of the throat are a problem in individual patients. Some patients who snore may require combined UPPP throat surgery and nasal surgery. This often increases the success rate in reducing snoring. One study that indicates the typical success rate from combining operations is that of Drs. J. Pichet and N. Gagnon of the University of Montreal Medical School in Canada. They sent a questionnaire regarding snoring to 180 patients who had UPPP plus nasal surgery, and 97 percent of them reported that their snoring had improved.

In most hospitals, the success rate of UPPP as a treatment for snoring is about 85 to 90 percent of patients. Failures most often occur in patients who are overweight. The success rate of the procedure as a treatment for sleep apnea is lower—UPPP is successful in reducing or eliminating apnea in only about 50 percent of cases. For severe apnea, it seldom is successful at all.

One reason for failures is that the obstruction in the throat causing the sleep apnea occurs at a level in the airway that is not accessible to the surgeon. For example, if the obstruction occurs behind the tongue or lower in the throat, UPPP will not be successful.

Another thing that makes it difficult to predict success of the treatment is that in many patients, obstruction may occur at several places along the airway, so that even if surgery is performed well at one location, the airway may still be obstructed at another location, so that snoring and apnea may continue. Dr. O. Skatvedt of the department of otolaryngology at Ullevaal University Hospital in Oslo, Norway, showed this in a study of twenty patients, all of whom were snorers and most of whom had sleep apnea. Dr. Skatvedt used sophisticated techniques to identify the sites of obstruction and found that of the twenty patients, thirteen had obstruction in two or more segments of the airway.

So if you decide to have surgery, and afterward find out that you still have snoring and sleep apnea, it is most likely not the surgeon's fault, but is a result of having obstruction at a location within the airway that the surgeon could not access or an obstruction at a second location that was unknown.

Other Anatomical Conditions That Sometimes Cause Snoring

There are some other conditions that can cause snoring and can be treated by surgery, but they are more rare. These surgical approaches do not involve operation on the uvula or soft palate, but involve other structures. These approaches are more complex, but not necessarily any more dangerous, than UPPP. They have only been performed in patients with sleep apnea, but because snoring almost invariably accompanies sleep apnea, the operations, if successful, will usually also cure snoring.

For example, some people have a receding chin that impedes efficient airflow. Although surgery designed to correct this abnormality is more complex than removing tonsils, polyps, or adenoids, it is usually quite successful in resolving snoring and apnea.

The goal of these surgeries is to enlarge the airway. The first step is to advance the tongue forward, without disturbing the position of the upper and lower jaw. This procedure is called *genioglossal advancement with hyoid myotomy (GAHM)*. The next step, if needed, is more complex: to advance both jaws. This is called *maxillo-mandibular osteotomy (MMO)*. Although the airway can be enlarged by advancing only the lower jaw, the upper one must also be advanced in order not to disturb the bite. Most of the time patients who reach the point of needing these procedures have already had UPPP without success. In carefully selected patients, these procedures can be successful in getting rid of apnea (and hopefully snoring), but they are not routinely recommended for treatment of nonapneic snoring.

Other conditions can narrow the airway, too. For example, an enlarged thyroid closed one patient's airway to the size of a pencil. Surgery solved the problem. Sometimes extensive liposuction of tissues around the neck is tried, but results have not been outstanding.

Laser Surgery

Laser-assisted uvulopalatoplasty (LAUP) is a surgical procedure that involves partial removal of the uvula and soft palate using a laser. It is a simpler procedure than UPPP to treat snoring, and can be done on an outpatient basis.

A laser is an instrument that produces a beam of light strong enough to cut through tissue (or steel when used in industry). It usually seals blood vessels as it cuts and so minimizes bleeding. Lasers used as scalpels in medicine are usually pulsed to prevent heat buildup and injury to tissue.

LAUP differs from conventional UPPP in several respects. First, the cutting tool is different—a laser is used instead of a scalpel or electrocautery. Second, there is less removal of tissues—only parts of the uvula and extra tissue of the soft palate are removed, but the tonsils and the sides of the throat (called the pharynx) are not operated on as they are in UPPP (although some surgeons will try to modify the pharynx somewhat). Third, the setting is different—LAUP is usually done in the office, in several stages; if snoring persists, surgery is repeated, removing more tissue each time. Fourth, the anesthesia procedure is different—laser surgery is usually carried out under a local anesthetic, much like what you get when you go to the dentist, whereas UPPP is usually done in the hospital under a general anesthetic.

The LAUP technique involves removing the edges of the soft palate and then shortening and reshaping the uvula to give more space to the crowded airway and to eliminate tissues likely to vibrate. During healing, scar tissue forms around the uvula and palate, stiffening these structures while also increasing the antisnoring effect.

LAUP was first described in 1990 by Dr. Yves-Victor Kamami of the department of otorhinolaryngology at the Foch Hospital in Paris, France. Between 1988 and 1990 he operated on thirty-one patients and reported that after two to seven sessions (an average of four sessions) in twenty-four of them, snoring was either completely eliminated or was no longer disturbing to the bedpartner. It is not clear from his description whether sleep studies were done before and after surgery, how long after surgery the patients were asked about their snoring, or whether snoring had changed or returned at later follow-up. By 1994 Dr. Kamami had operated on 741 patients and reported a 95 percent success rate and no serious complications.

In the United States, Dr. Yosef Krespi and colleagues of the department of otolaryngology at St. Luke's/Roosevelt Hospital Center at Columbia University in New York City reported on a study of 307 patients who were treated with LAUP for their snoring. The cure rate (i.e., snoring was eliminated) was 84 percent, with an additional 7 percent reporting improvement of snoring. Long-term results were not given, although there were some patients who were followed for up to two years.

But not all surgeons have had a high success rate with LAUP for treatment of snoring. For example, Dr. Takehiro Hanada and colleagues in the department of otorhinolaryngology at the Kagoshima University in Kagoshima, Japan, found only about a 50 percent success rate in 106 patients treated with LAUP for snoring.

There could be many reasons for the differences—it is difficult to compare various studies dealing with the effectiveness of LAUP because the surgical approaches are not precisely the same, resulting in different degrees of tissue modification, and the number of surgical procedures differs in various studies. Some surgeons perform LAUP as a single-stage procedure, others do sequential modification in up to seven sessions. Comparisons are also difficult because follow-up times are short, the grading of snoring is not standardized, and sleep studies are not usually done before and after surgery.

We report this information to you in so much detail because we want you to understand that opinions on the techniques and degrees of success vary. If you're contemplating surgery, we want you to be as informed as possible as you and your surgeon work together to reach a decision.

The side effects of LAUP are not yet well established, particularly long-term side effects, but they appear to be about the same as with UPPP. There often is pain that persists for several weeks after surgery. There can occasionally be scarring and narrowing of the throat that interferes permanently with swallowing and speech. It is also possible that LAUP, like UPPP, may mask sleep apnea by altering or removing the snoring that otherwise serves as a warning signal for apnea. So the bottom line is that LAUP and UPPP are equal as far as side effects and success rates are concerned. And of course, LAUP is less expensive since it does not require hospitalization.

At the University of Toronto, where we have performed surgeries on hundreds of patients, we have found that of patients who have UPPP for snoring, in about 50 percent snoring is eliminated, and in about 80 percent it is reduced. This is determined by questioning patients and their bedpartners after surgery. Of patients having LAUP the success rate is 80 to 90 percent, the same rate reported by most surgeons today.

Today there is no reason to have a UPPP only for restructuring or removal of the uvula or soft palate. The LAUP, an outpatient laser procedure, would be the procedure of choice. In most cases, the only reason for UPPP is that enlarged tonsils are also to be removed or more extensive areas of the throat are to be operated on.

The Newest Technique: Surgery by Radio-Frequency Energy

A new surgical treatment has just been developed that may improve the picture of surgical treatment of snoring and apnea. It is still being tested. The technique, called *somnoplasty*, uses radio-frequency energy to shrink the tissues that block the airway.

A radio-frequency generator is connected to a narrow needle that is used to apply low-power radio waves to problem tissues in the inner nose or at the base of the tongue, or to the uvula or other parts of the throat or soft palate. The radio waves destroy whatever excess tissue is blocking the airway and causing the snoring problem. The physician can choose one area to do the procedure on or a combination of areas, depending on which areas are causing the problem. Sometimes a second treatment is done later to extend the area treated.

The radio waves destroy small areas of tissue by heating the tissue. However, the temperatures are not high, only about 10 percent of the temperatures achieved during laser surgery. This results in much less heat being created in surrounding tissues and much less damage to them. The small needle used in the technique allows very precise targeting of the tissue.

The scar tissue that is formed is then resorbed by the body after a few weeks, resulting in reduced size of the tissue blocking the airway and a more open airway. Also tissue in the area tends to contract and stiffen, which reduces its tendency to vibrate.

The major advantages of this technique over UPPP or LAUP are that surgery is more localized and the tissues are not cut. Therefore, there is less damage to the throat, less bleeding, less pain, fewer complications, and a shorter recovery time. The procedure is simple—it takes less than a half hour in the office—and can be performed as an outpatient procedure using topical or local anesthesia. Another advantage is that it may be possible to shape the energy-delivering needle in such a way as to access the tissues behind and below the tongue—something that cannot be done presently with scalpel or laser.

In the first study reported (May 1998) in 22 patients who had the procedure done for snoring, the procedure was shown to be safe and essentially painless and reduced snoring significantly. Patients had a sore throat, but only half required simple medication for pain, and usually only for one to three days. Snoring usually became worse for a time until the tissue swelling went down.

The developer of the technique and the instrumentation is Somnus Medical Technologies, hence the name "somnoplasty" for the procedure.

The procedure is being evaluated in many universities and hospitals around the world, but as yet there are no data to determine whether this technique will have any better success rate than UPPP or LAUP. The reports so far indicate an encouraging success rate in eliminating or lessening snoring.

Making the Decision

It is easy to understand why surgery is attractive to the person whose snoring is so bad the bedpartner cannot stay in the same room. It offers the possibility of a permanent cure.

However, before you decide to have any of the surgeries for snoring, you must remember that without modifying other risk factors, such as obesity, alcohol, smoking, or allergies, it is unlikely that you will be cured.

If you are considering LAUP, you should know that although LAUP may work for serious snoring, the American Sleep Disorders Association does not recommend it for treatment of sleep apnea. The results are not as good for apnea as for snoring, and some physicians worry that without the snoring a bedpartner might not awake and thus never become aware of the apnea. The ASDA recommends that patients undergoing LAUP have a sleep study before surgery to see whether they have sleep apnea.

Deciding whether to have surgery is not easy. Many questions are still unanswered, and we still do not have significant documentation as to its long-term effectiveness over the years following surgery. We do know that the best surgical candidate is a person who is not overweight and does not have apnea. However, surgery in the throat area can change the voice and airstream, so it may be chancy for a professional singer, actor, or wind instrument player to have this surgery.

Since snoring affects the family, you should bring your spouse along to preliminary consultations as you make your decision. Discuss the pros and cons with your doctor, and ask for advice regarding which surgery to perform in your particular case. If you are contemplating surgery, make sure that you work with your doctor to choose a surgeon who has experience and up-to-date knowledge of the procedure that will be used.

By the way, anyone with sleep apnea who is scheduled for *any* kind of surgery should be sure that the anesthesiologist is aware of the apnea so that preoperative sedation will be minimal, an appropriate anesthetic agent will be used, and special arrangements will be made for postoperative monitoring, including having CPAP on hand. Your surgeon and your anesthesiologist, once they are aware of the severity of your apnea, will decide on the best type of anesthesia for you—usually a regional anesthesia such as an epidural, spinal, or peripheral nerve block rather than general anesthesia.

Here are some questions you may wish to ask the surgeon as you consider your decision:

- Given your throat anatomy and the results of tests, are you a good candidate for surgical success?
- How much training and experience does the surgeon have in the procedure that you would be having? What is the surgeon's success rate?
- Would any of your other health conditions make the surgery inappropriate?
- Will the surgery require general or local anesthesia?
- What is the estimated recovery time? How long will you be away from work?
- What are the possible side effects?
- How much will the procedure cost? Will it be covered by insurance?

Before you have surgery we recommend that you see a sleep disorders specialist who can arrange for preoperative evaluation to determine the cause or causes of your snoring. After all, if your snoring is caused by a broken nose, operating on your uvula isn't going to help. Then make your decision in consultation with a medical specialist and act on those recommendations.

After surgery, you should have regular follow-up appointments to determine the success of the surgery and to monitor for possible post-operative complications. Sometimes medications for other conditions will also need to be adjusted; with improvement in snoring and apnea, for example, high blood pressure may decrease so that you might need less medicine or a different, less strong medicine for it.

And remember that even though your snoring may be cured, you should in the future still be on the look out for apnea. If it occurs, or if you start experiencing snoring or excessive daytime sleepiness again, you should check back with a sleep specialist.

Even if you decide to have surgery, we recommend that before the surgery you carry out the noninvasive approaches in our no-more-snoring program outlined in chapters 4 through 8. Taking steps to reduce your risk factors will increase your chances of a successful surgery. In fact, in some cases, lifestyle changes and reducing weight can be so successful in combating the snoring that it will make the surgery unnecessary.

If you have surgery, after the surgery do not gain weight or fall back into any lifestyle habits that are factors in causing snoring. If you gain a substantial amount of weight after corrective surgery, you can defeat the benefits of the surgery and start snoring again.

Maintain our no-more-snoring program and it will increase your chances of having peaceful snore-free nights and great fatigue-free days. That is what we wish for you—good nights and wonderful days.

Appendix A

Sleep Disorders Centers and Laboratories

Sleep Disorders Centers and Laboratories in the United States

The following sleep disorders centers and laboratories are accredited members of the American Sleep Disorders Association. Some are laboratories accredited only for the diagnosis and treatment of sleep-related breathing disorders. Others are sleep disorders centers, accredited for the diagnosis and treatment of all types of disorders of sleep and alertness.

The list is updated periodically. You can obtain a current listing or other information about sleep disorders from the American Sleep Disorders Association, 1610 Fourteenth Street NW, Rochester, MN 55901, or visit the ASDA web site (www.asda.org).

ALABAMA

Breathing Disorders Lab
Athens-Limestone Hospital
Athens, AL 35612
256-233-9473

Sleep Disorders Center
Brookwood Medical Center
2010 Brookwood Medical Center Drive
Birmingham, AL 35209
205-877-2486, fax: 205-877-1663

Sleep Disorders Center of Alabama
790 Montclair Road
Birmingham, AL 35213
205-599-1020, fax: 205-599-1029

Sleep-Wake Disorders Center
University of Alabama–Birmingham
1713 Sixth Avenue South
Birmingham, AL 35233
205-934-7110

Sleep Disorder Lab
Carraway Methodist Medical Center
Birmingham, AL 35234
202-502-6164

Sleep Disorders Center
Marshall Medical Center
Boaz, AL 35957
205-593-1226

Sleep Disorders Center
Huntington Memorial Hospital
Pasadena, CA 91109
818-397-3061

Sleep Disorders Center
Doctors Medical Center–Pinole
2151 Appian Way
Pinole, CA 94564
510-741-2525 or 800-640-9440

Sleep Disorders Center
Pomona Valley Hospital Medical Center
1798 North Garey Avenue
Pomona, CA 91767
909-865-9587, fax: 909-865-9969

Center for Sleep Apnea
Redding Medical Center
2801 Eureka Way
Redding, CA 96001
916-245-4187, fax: 916-245-4116

Sequoia Sleep Disorders Center
Sequoia Hospital
Redwood City, CA 94062
650-367-5137, fax: 650-363-5304

Sutter Sleep Disorders Center
650 Howe Avenue
Sacramento, CA 95825
916-646-3300

Sleep Disorders Center
University of California Davis Medical
    Center
2315 Stockton Boulevard
Sacramento, CA 95817
916-734-0256, fax: 916-452-2739

Inland Sleep Center
401 East Highland Avenue
San Bernardino, CA 92404
909-883-8058

Mercy Sleep Disorders Center
Mercy-Scripps Health
4077 Fifth Avenue
San Diego, CA 92103
619-260-7378, fax: 619-686-3990

San Diego Sleep Disorders Center
1842 Third Avenue
San Diego, CA 92101
619-235-0248

Stanford Health Services Sleep Clinic
2340 Clay Street
San Francisco, CA 94115
415-923-3336, fax: 415-923-3584

UCSF/Stanford Sleep Disorders Center
University of California–San Francisco
1600 Divisadero Street
San Francisco, CA 94115
415-885-7886, fax: 415-885-3650

Sleep Disorders Center of Santa Barbara
2410 Fletcher Avenue
Santa Barbara, CA 93105
805-898-8845, fax: 805-898-8848

Sleep Disorders Clinic
Stanford University Medical Center
401 Quarry Road
Stanford, CA 94305
415-723-6601, fax: 415-725-8910

Southern California Sleep Apnea Center
Lombard Medical Group
2230 Lynn Road
Thousand Oaks, CA 91360
805-495-1066, fax: 805-497-1782

Torrance Memorial Medical Center
Sleep Disorders Center
3330 West Lomita Boulevard
Torrance, CA 90505
310-517-4617, fax: 310-784-4869

Sleep Disorders Laboratory
Kaweah Delta District Hospital
Visalia, CA 93291
209-625-7338, fax: 209-635-4059

West Valley Sleep Disorders Center
7320 Woodlake Avenue
West Hills, CA 91307
818-715-0096, fax: 818-716-1875

Sleep Disorders Center
Woodland Memorial Hospital
Woodland, CA 95695
916-668-2695, fax: 916-668-5787

COLORADO

National Jewish/University of Colorado
  Sleep Center
1400 Jackson Street
Denver, CO 80206
303-398-1523

Sleep Disorders Center
Columbia Presbyerian St. Luke's Medical
  Center
Denver, CO 80218
303-839-6049

Sleep Center of Southern Colorado
Parkview Medical Center
400 West Sixteenth Street
Pueblo, CO 81003
719-584-4659, fax: 719-584-4929

CONNECTICUT

Sleep Disorders Center
Danbury Hospital
Danbury, CT 06810
203-731-8033, fax: 203-731-8628

Gaylord-Yale Sleep Disorders
  Laboratory
Gaylord Hospital
Wallingford, CT 06492
203-284-2853

DELAWARE

Sleep Disorders Center
Christiana Hospital
Newark, DE 19718
302-478-4600

Sleep Disorders Center
Christiana Health Services
Wilmington, DE 19899
302-478-4600

DISTRICT OF COLUMBIA

Sleep Disorders Center
Sibley Memorial Hospital
Washington, DC 20016
202-364-7676, fax: 202-362-9378

Sleep Disorders Center
Georgetown University Hospital
Washington, DC 20007
202-784-3610, fax: 202-784-2920

FLORIDA

Boca Raton Sleep Disorders Center
899 Meadows Road
Boca Raton, FL 33486
561-750-9881, fax: 561-750-9644

Sleep Disorder Laboratory
Broward General Medical Center
1600 South Andrews Avenue
Fort Lauderdale, FL 33316
954-355-5534

Mayo Sleep Disorders Center
Mayo Clinic Jacksonville
4500 San Pablo Road
Jacksonville, FL 32224
904-953-7287, fax: 904-953-7388

Watson Clinic Sleep Disorders Center
1600 Lakeland Hills Boulevard
Lakeland, FL 33804
941-680-7627, fax: 941-680-7430

Atlantic Sleep Disorders Center
1401 South Apollo Boulevard
Melbourne, FL 32901
407-952-5191

Sleep Disorders Center
Miami Children's Hospital
Miami, FL 33155
305-662-8330

Sleep Disorders Center
University of Miami School of Medicine
Miami, FL 33101
305-324-3371

Sleep Disorders Center
Mount Sinai Medical Center
Miami Beach, FL 33140
305-674-2613

Munroe Regional Medical Center Sleep
  Laboratory
131 SW Fifteenth Street
Ocala, FL 34473
352-351-7279, fax: 352-351-7280

Florida Hospital Sleep Disorders Center
601 East Rollins Avenue
Orlando, FL 32803
407-897-1558, fax: 407-897-1775

Health First Sleep Disorders Center
Palm Bay Community Hospital
Palm Bay, FL 32907
407-722-8087, fax: 407-722-8496

Sleep Disorders Center
West Florida Medical Center
Pensacola, FL 32514
850-494-4850

St. Petersburg Sleep Disorders Center
2525 Pasadena Avenue South
St. Petersburg, FL 33707
813-360-0853 or 800-242-3244 (in
  Florida)

Sleep Disorders Center
Sarasota Memorial Hospital
Sarasota, FL 34239
941-917-2525, fax: 941-917-6187

Tallahassee Sleep Disorders Center
1304 Hodges Drive
Tallahassee, FL 32308
800-662-4278 or 904-681-5800

Laboratory for Sleep Related Breathing
  Disorders
University Community Hospital
Tampa, FL 33613
813-979-7410, fax: 813-632-7517

GEORGIA

Atlanta Center for Sleep Disorders
303 Parkway Drive
Atlanta, GA 30312
404-265-3722, fax: 404-265-3833

Sleep Disorders Center
Northside Hospital
Atlanta, GA 30342
404-851-8135, fax: 404-252-9946

Sleep Disorders Center of Georgia
5505 Peachtree Dunwoody Road
Atlanta, GA 30342
404-257-0080, fax: 404-257-0592

Central Georgia Sleep Disorders Center
777 Hemlock Street
Macon, GA 31202
912-633-7222, fax: 912-745-5125

Sleep Disorders Center
Promina Kennestone Hospital
Marietta, GA 30060
770-793-5353, fax: 770-793-5357

Sleep Disorders Medicine Candler
  Hospital
Savannah, GA 31405
912-692-6673, fax: 912-692-6931

Savannah Sleep Disorders Center
St. Joseph's Hospital
Savannah, GA 31419
912-927-5141, fax: 912-921-3380

Sleep Disorders Center
Memorial Medical Center
Savannah, GA 31403
912-350-8327

HAWAII

Orchid Isle Sleep Lab
1404 Kilauea Avenue
Hilo, HI 96743
808-935-6105

Pulmonary Sleep Disorders Center
Kuakini Medical Center
347 North Kuakini Street
Honolulu, HI 96817
808-547-9119, fax: 808-547-9225

Sleep Laboratory
Queen's Medical Center
Honolulu, HI 96813
808-547-4396

Sleep Disorders Center of the Pacific
Straub Clinic and Hospital
Honolulu, HI 96813
808-522-4448, fax: 808-522-3048

Orchid Isles Respiratory Services
Waimes Town Plaza
Kamuela, HI 96743
808-885-7351

IDAHO

Idaho Sleep Disorders Laboratory
St. Luke's Regional Medical Center
Boise, ID 83712
208-381-2440

Idaho Diagnostic Sleep Lab
526-C Shoup Avenue West
Twin Falls, ID 83301
208-736-7646

ILLINOIS

Center for Sleep and Ventilatory
    Disorders
University of Illinois–Chicago
1740 West Taylor Street
Chicago, IL 60612
312-996-7708

Sleep Disorders Center
Northwestern Memorial Hospital
303 East Superior
Chicago, IL 60611
312-908-8120 or 312-908-8508

Sleep Disorders Center
University of Chicago Hospitals
5841 South Maryland
Chicago, IL 60637
773-702-1782, fax: 773-702-7998

Sleep Disorder Service and Research
    Center
Rush-Presbyterian–St. Luke's Medical
    Center
Chicago, IL 60612
312-942-5440, fax: 312-942-4990

Sleep Disorders Center
Evanston Hospital
Evanston, IL 60201
847-570-2567, fax: 847-570-2984

Sleep Disorders Center
Lutheran General Hospital
Park Ridge, IL 60068
847-723-7024, fax: 847-723-7369

C. Duane Morgan Sleep Disorders
    Center
Methodist Medical Center of Illinois
221 NE Glen Oak Avenue
Peoria, IL 61636
309-672-4966 or 309-671-5136

Sleep Disorders Lab
Rochford Health System
Rockford, IL 61103
815-971-5595

Sleep Disorders Center
SIU School of Medicine/Memorial
    Medical Center
800 North Rutledge
Springfield, IL 62781
217-788-4269

Carle Regional Sleep Disorders Center
Carle Foundation Hospital
Urbana, IL 61801
217-383-3364

Sleep Disorders Center
Central DuPage Hospital
Winfield, IL 60190
630-682-1600

INDIANA

Sleep Disorders Center
St. Francis Hospital and Health Centers
1500 Albany Street
Beech Grove, IN 46107
317-783-8144, fax: 317-781-1402

St. Mary's Sleep Disorders Center
St. Mary's Medical Center
3700 Washington Avenue
Evansville, IN 47750
812-485-4960, fax: 812-485-7953

St. Joseph Sleep Disorders Center
St. Joseph Medical Center
700 Broadway
Fort Wayne, IN 46802
219-425-3552

Sleep/Wake Disorders Center
Community Hospitals of Indianapolis
1500 North Ritter Avenue
Indianapolis, IN 46219
317-355-4275, fax: 317-351-2785

Sleep Disorders Center
St. Vincent Hospital
Indianapolis, IN 46260
317-338-2152

Sleep/Wake Disorders Center
Winona Memorial Hospital
Indianapolis, IN 46208
317-927-2100

Sleep Alertness Center
Lafayette Home Hospital
Lafayette, IN 47904
317-447-6811

IOWA

Sleep Disorders Center
Mary Greeley Medical Center
Ames, IA 50010
515-239-2353

Sleep Disorders Center
University of Iowa Hospitals and Clinics
Iowa City, IA 52242
319-356-3813, fax: 319-356-4505

KANSAS

Sleep Disorders Center
St. Francis Hospital and Medical Center
Topeka, KS 66606
913-295-7900

Sleep Disorders Center
Wesley Medical Center
550 North Hillside
Wichita, KS 67214
316-688-2663, fax: 316-688-3256

KENTUCKY

Sleep Diagnostics Lab
Columbia/Greenview Regional Hospital
1801 Ashley Circle
Bowling Green, KY 42101
502-793-2175, fax: 502-793-2177

Sleep Lab
Medical Center at Bowling Green
250 Park Street
Bowling Green, KY 42101
502-745-1024

Physicians' Center for Sleep Disorders
Graves-Gilbert Clinic
201 Park Street
Bowling Green, KY 42102
502-781-5111

Sleep Disorders Center
St. Luke Hospital
Florence, KY 41042
606-525-5347, fax: 606-572-3375

The Sleep Disorder Center
St. Luke Hospital
Fort Thomas, KY 41075
606-572-3535

Sleep Apnea Center
Jennie Stuart Medical Center
Hopkinsville, KY 42240
502-887-0412

Sleep Apnea Center
Samaritan Hospital
310 South Limestone
Lexington, KY 40508
606-252-6612, fax: 606-252-6612

Sleep Disorders Center
St. Joseph's Hospital
Lexington, KY 40504
606-278-0444

Caritas Sleep Apnea Center
Caritas Medical Center
1850 Bluegrass Avenue
Louisville, KY 40215
502-361-6555

Sleep Disorders Center
Columbia Audubon Hospital
Louisville, KY 40217
502-636-7459

Sleep Disorders Center
University of Louisville Hospital
Louisville, KY 40202
502-562-3792, fax: 502-562-4632

Sleep Medicine Specialists
1169 Eastern Parkway
Louisville, KY 40217
502-454-0755, fax: 502-454-3497

Regional Medical Center Lab for Sleep-
   Related Breathing Disorders
900 Hospital Drive
Madisonville, KY 42431
502-825-5918

Diller Regional Sleep Disorders Center
Lourdes Hospital
Paducah, KY 42001
502-444-2660, fax: 502-444-2661

Breathing Disorders Sleep Lab
Pikeville Methodist Hospital
Pikeville, KY 41501
606-437-3989, fax: 606-437-9649

Sleep Disorders Lab
PAC Hospital
Richmond, KY 40475
606-625-3334

LOUISIANA

Sleep Disorders Center
Memorial Medical Center
2700 Napoleon Avenue
New Orleans, LA 70115
504-896-5439, fax: 504-897-4403

Tulane Sleep Disorders Center
1415 Tulane Avenue
New Orleans, LA 70112
504-588-5231, fax: 504-584-1727

Sleep Disorders Center
LSU Medical Center
Shreveport, LA 71130
318-675-5365, fax: 318-675-4440

Neurology and Sleep Clinic
2205 East Seventieth Street
Shreveport, LA 71105
318-797-1585, fax: 318-797-6077

Sleep Disorders Center
North Shore Regional Medical Center
100 Medical Center Drive
Slidell, LA 70461
504-646-5711, fax: 504-646-5013

MAINE

Sleep Disorders Laboratory
St. Mary's Regional Medical Center
97 Campus Avenue
Lewiston, ME 04240
207-777-8959

Maine Institute for Sleep Breathing
   Disorders
930 Congress Street
Portland, ME 04102
207-871-4535

MARYLAND

Sleep Disorders Center
Johns Hopkins Bayview Medical Center
5501 Hopkins Bayview Circle
Baltimore, MD 21224
410-550-0571, fax: 410-550-3374

Maryland Sleep Disorders Center
Greater Baltimore Medical Center
6701 North Charles Street
Baltimore, MD 21204
410-494-9773, fax: 410-823-6635

Sleep Disorders Center
Frederick Memorial Hospital
Frederick, MD 21701
301-698-3802

Sleep-Breathing Disorders Center of
    Hagerstown
12821 Oak Hill Avenue
Hagerstown, MD 21742
301-733-5971

Shady Grove Sleep Disorders
    Center
14915 Broschart Road
Rockville, MD 20850
301-251-5905, fax: 301-251-6189

Washington Adventist Sleep Disorders
    Center
7525 Carroll Avenue
Takoma Park, MD 20912
301-891-2594

MASSACHUSETTS

Sleep Disorders Center
Beth Israel Deaconess Medical
    Center
330 Brookline Avenue
Boston, MA 02215
617-667-3237, fax: 617-667-5216

Sleep Disorders Center
Lahey-Hitchcock Clinic
41 Mall Road
Burlington, MA 01805
781-744-8251, fax: 781-744-5243

Sleep Disorders Institute of Central New
    England
St. Vincent Hospital
Worcester, MA 01604
508-798-6212, fax: 508-798-1121

MICHIGAN

Sleep Disorders Center
St. Joseph Mercy Hospital
Ann Arbor, MI 48106
313-712-4651

Sleep Disorders Center
University of Michigan Hospitals
1500 East Medical Center Drive
Ann Arbor, MI 48109
313-936-9068, fax: 313-936-5377

Sleep Disorders Clinic
Bay Medical Center
1900 Columbus Avenue
Bay City, MI 48708
517-894-3332, fax: 517-894-6114

Harper Hospital Sleep Disorders Center
4160 John R Street
Detroit, MI 48201
313-745-9009, fax: 313-745-8725

Sinai Sleep Center
Sinai Hospital
Detroit, MI 48235
313-493-5148

Sleep/Wake Disorders Laboratory
VA Medical Center
4646 John R Street
Detroit, MI 48201
313-576-1000

West Michigan Sleep Disorders Center
Butterworth Hospital
Grand Rapids, MI 49503
616-391-3759, fax: 616-391-3052

Sleep Disorders Center
Borgess Medical Center
1521 Gull Road
Kalamazoo, MI 49001
616-226-7081, fax: 616-226-6909

Sleep/Wake Center
Ingham Regional Medical Center
2025 South Washington Avenue
Lansing, MI 48910
517-372-6444, fax: 517-372-6440

Sparrow Sleep Center
Sparrow Hospital
Lansing, MI 48909
517-483-2946, fax: 517-483-2472

Sleep and Respiratory Associates of
 Michigan
28200 Franklin Road
Southfield, MI 48034
248-350-2722, fax: 248-350-0154

Munson Sleep Disorders Center
Munson Medical Center
1105 Sixth Street
Traverse City, MI 49684
800-358-9641 or 616-935-6600

Sleep Disorders Institute
44199 Dequindre
Troy, MI 48098
248-879-0707, fax: 248-879-2704

MINNESOTA

Duluth Regional Sleep Disorders
 Center
St. Mary's Medical Center
407 East Third Street
Duluth, MN 55805
218-726-4692

Fairview Sleep Center
Fairview Southdale Hospital
Edina, MN 55435
612-924-5053

Minnesota Regional Sleep Disorders
 Center
Hennepin County Medical Center
701 Park Avenue South
Minneapolis, MN 55415
612-347-6288, fax: 612-904-4207

Sleep Disorders Center
Abbott Northwestern Hospital
800 East Twenty-eighth Street at Chicago
 Avenue
Minneapolis, MN 55407
612-863-4516, fax: 612-863-2837

Mayo Sleep Disorders Center
Mayo Clinic
200 First Street SW
Rochester, MN 55905
507-266-8900, fax: 507-266-7772

Sleep Disorders Center
Methodist Hospital
St. Louis Park, MN 55426
612-993-6083, fax: 612-993-5069

Sleep Diagnostic Center
St. Joseph's Hospital
69 West Exchange Street
St. Paul, MN 55102
612-232-3682, fax: 612-232-4111

MISSISSIPPI

Sleep Disorders Center
Memorial Hospital at Gulfport
Gulfport, MS 39501
601-865-3152, fax: 601-865-3259

Sleep Disorders Center
Forrest General Hospital
Hattiesburg, MS 39401
601-288-4790 or 800-280-8520

Sleep Disorders Center
University of Mississippi Medical
 Center
2500 North State Street
Jackson, MS 39216
601-984-4820, fax: 601-984-5885

MISSOURI

Unity Sleep Medicine and Research
 Center
St. Luke's Hospital
Chesterfield, MO 63017
314-205-6030, fax: 314-205-6025

University of Missouri Sleep Disorders
 Center
University Hospital and Clinics
One Hospital Drive
Columbia, MO 65212
573-884-SLEEP or 800-ADD-SLEEP, fax:
 573-884-4785

Sleep Disorders Center
Research Medical Center
2316 East Meyer Boulevard
Kansas City, MO 64132
816-276-4334, fax: 816-276-3488

Sleep Disorders Center
St. Luke's Hospital
4400 Wornall Road
Kansas City, MO 64111
816-932-3207

Sleep Disorders and Research Center
Deaconess Medical Center
6150 Oakland Avenue
St. Louis, MO 63139
314-768-3100, fax: 314-768-3594

Sleep Disorders Center
Health Services Division of St. Louis
   University
1221 South Grand Boulevard
St. Louis, MO 63104
314-577-8705, fax: 314-664-7248

Cox Regional Sleep Disorders
   Center
3800 South National Avenue
Springfield, MO 65807
417-269-5575, fax: 417-269-5578

Sleep Disorders Center
St. John's Regional Health Center
1235 East Cherokee
Springfield, MO 65804
417-885-5464, fax: 417-885-5465

MONTANA

Sleep Disorders Center
Deaconess Billings Clinic
2800 Tenth Avenue North
Billings, MT 59107
406-657-4075, fax: 406-657-4717

Sleep Center
St. Vincent Hospital
Billings, MT 59101
406-238-6815

NEBRASKA

Breathing Disorders Lab
Bryan Memorial Hospital
Lincoln, NE 68506
402-483-3950

Great Plains Regional Sleep Physiology
   Center
Lincoln General Hospital
Lincoln, NE 68502
402-473-5338, fax: 402-473-5380

Sleep Disorders Center
Clarkson Hospital
Omaha, NE 68105
402-552-2286, fax: 402-552-2057

Sleep Disorders Center
Methodist/Richard Young Hospital
Omaha, NE 68105
402-354-6305 or 402-354-6309

NEVADA

Sleep Clinic of Nevada
1012 East Sahara Avenue
Las Vegas, NV 89104
702-893-0020, fax: 702-893-0025

Washoe Sleep Disorders Center and
   Sleep Laboratory
Washoe Medical Center
75 Pringle Way
Reno, NV 89502
702-328-4700 or 800-JETLAGG

NEW HAMPSHIRE

Sleep Disorders Center
Dartmouth-Hitchcock Medical
   Center
One Medical Center Drive
Lebanon, NH 03756
603-650-7534, fax: 603-650-7820

Center for Sleep Evaluation
Catholic Medical Center
100 McGregor Street
Manchester, NH 03102
603-663-6680, fax: 603-663-6699

NEW JERSEY

SleepCare Center
457 Haddonfield Road
Cherry Hill, NJ 08002
609-662-5001, fax: 609-662-5187

Institute for Sleep/Wake Disorders
Hackensack University Medical Center
385 Prospect Avenue
Hackensack, NJ 07601
201-996-2992

Sleep Disorder Center
Morristown Memorial Hospital
Morristown, NJ 07962
973-971-4567, fax: 973-290-7620

Sleep Disorders Center
Memorial Hospital of Burlington County
Mount Holly, NJ 08060
609-267-0700, fax: 609-261-8619

Comprehensive Sleep Disorders Center
Robert Wood Johnson University
    Hospital
New Brunswick, NJ 08903
908-937-8683, fax: 908-418-8448

Sleep Disorders Center
Newark Beth Israel Medical Center
201 Lyons Avenue
Newark, NJ 07112
201-926-6668, fax: 201-923-6672

Sleep Disorders Center
Mercer Medical Center
446 Bellevue Avenue
Trenton, NJ 08607
609-394-4167, fax: 609-394-4352

Snoring and Sleep Apnea Center
Helene Fuld Medical Center
750 Brunswick Avenue
Trenton, NJ 08638
609-278-6990, fax: 609-278-6982

Sleep Disorders Center
2253 South Avenue
Westfield, NJ 07090
908-789-4244

NEW MEXICO

Sleep Disorders Center
Lovelace Health Systems
2929 Coors Road NW
Albuquerque, NM 87102
505-839-2369

University Hospital Sleep Disorders
    Center
4775 Indian School Road NE
Albuquerque, NM 87110
505-272-6101, fax: 505-272-6112

NEW YORK

Capital Region Sleep/Wake Disorders
    Center
St. Peter's Hospital and Albany Medical
    Center
25 Hackett Boulevard
Albany, NY 12208
518-436-9253

Bronx Sleep-Wake Disorders Center
Montefiore Medical Center
111 East 210th Street
Bronx, NY 10467
718-920-4841, fax: 718-798-4352

Health Care Sleep Disorders Center
1 Atwell Street
Cooperstown, NY 13326
607-547-6979

Sleep Disorders Center
St. Joseph's Hospital
Elmira, NY 14902
607-737-7008

Sleep Disorders Center
Winthrop-University Hospital
Mineola, NY 11501
516-663-3907, fax: 516-663-4788

Sleep-Wake Disorders Center
Long Island Jewish Medical Center
270-05 Seventy-sixth Avenue
New Hyde Park, NY 11042
718-470-7058

New York Hospital–Cornell Manhattan
Campus
520 East Seventieth Street
New York, NY 10021
914-997-5751

Sleep Disorders Center
Columbia-Presbyterian Medical Center
161 Fort Washington Avenue
New York, NY 10032
212-305-1860 or 914-948-0400

Sleep Disorders Institute
St. Luke's/Roosevelt Hospital Center
1090 Amsterdam Avenue
New York, NY 10025
212-523-1700, fax: 212-523-1704

Sleep Disorders Center of Rochester
2110 Clinton Avenue South
Rochester, NY 14618
716-442-4141, fax: 716-442-6259

Sleep Disorders Center
State University of New York–Stony Brook
Stony Brook, NY 11794
516-444-2916, fax: 516-444-7851

Sleep Center
Community General Hospital
Broad Road
Syracuse, NY 13215
315-492-5877, fax: 315-492-5521

Sleep Laboratory
St. Joseph's Hospital Health Center
945 East Genesee Street
Syracuse, NY 13210
315-475-3379

Sleep Disorders Center
St. Elizabeth Medical Center
Utica, NY 13501
315-734-3484

Sleep Disorders Center–White Plains
Columbia-Presbyterian Medical Center
185 Maple Avenue
White Plains, NY 10601
914-948-0595

Sleep-Wake Disorders Center
New York Hospital–Cornell Medical
Center
21 Bloomingdale Road
White Plains, NY 10605
914-997-5751, fax: 914-682-6911

NORTH CAROLINA

Sleep Medicine Center of Asheville
1091 Hendersonville Road
Asheville, NC 28803
828-277-7533, fax: 828-277-7493

Western Carolina Sleep Center
Mission/St. Joseph's Hospitals
Asheville, NC 28801
828-258-6708

Carolinas Sleep Services
University Hospital
Charlotte, NC 28256
704-548-5855, fax: 704-548-6848

Carolinas Sleep Services
Mercy Hospital South
Charlotte, NC 28210
704-543-2213

Sleep Disorders Center
Moses H. Cone Memorial Hospital
Greensboro, NC 27401
910-574-7406

Sleep Medicine Center of Salisbury
911 West Henderson Street
Salisbury, NC 28144
704-637-1533, fax: 704-637-0470

Sleep Disorders Center
North Carolina Baptist Hospital
Bowman Gray School of Medicine
Winston-Salem, NC 27157
910-716-5288

Sleep Disorders Center
160 Charlois Boulevard
Winston-Salem, NC 27103
910-765-9431, fax: 910-765-4889

OHIO

Sleep Disorders Center
Bethesda Oak Hospital
619 Oak Street
Cincinnati, OH 45206
513-569-6320, fax: 513-569-5495

Tri-State Sleep Disorders Center
1275 East Kemper Road
Cincinnati, OH 45246
513-671-3101

Cardiopulmonary Sleep Laboratory
15805 Puritas Avenue
Cleveland, OH 44135
216-267-5933, fax: 216-267-5133

Sleep Disorders Center
Cleveland Clinic Foundation
9500 Euclid Avenue
Cleveland, OH 44195
216-444-2165, fax: 216-445-4378

University Sleep Center
University Hospitals of Cleveland
11100 Euclid Avenue
Cleveland, OH 44106
216-844-1301

Sleep Disorders Center
Ohio State University Medical Center
410 West Tenth Avenue
Columbus, OH 43210
614-293-8296, fax: 614-293-4506

Center for Sleep and Wake Disorders
Miami Valley Hospital
Dayton, OH 45409
937-208-2515

Sleep Disorders Center
Good Samaritan Hospital
Dayton, OH 45406
937-276-8307

Ohio Sleep Medicine and Neuroscience
    Institute
4975 Bradenton Avenue
Dublin, OH 43017
614-766-0773, fax: 614-766-2599

Sleep Disorders Center
Kettering Medical Center
3535 Southern Boulevard
Kettering, OH 45429
937-296-7805, fax: 937-296-7821

Ohio Sleep Disorders Center
150 Springside Drive
Montrose, OH 44333
330-670-1290

Northwest Ohio Sleep Disorders Center
Toledo Hospital
Toledo, OH 43606
419-471-5629, fax: 419-479-6954

Sleep Disorders Center
St. Vincent Medical Center
2213 Cherry Street
Toledo, OH 43608
419-321-4980

Sleep Disorders Center
Good Samaritan Medical Center
800 Forest Avenue
Zanesville, OH 43701
614-454-5855, fax: 614-455-7645

OKLAHOMA

Sleep Disorders Center of Oklahoma
Integris Health
4401 South Western Avenue
Oklahoma City, OK 73109
405-636-7700

OREGON

Sleep Disorders Center
Sacred Heart Medical Center
1255 Hilyard Street
Eugene, OR 97440
503-686-7224

Sleep Disorders Center
Rogue Valley Medical Center
2825 East Barnett Road
Medford, OR 97504
541-608-4320, fax: 541-608-5890

Legacy Good Samaritan Sleep Disorders
Center
1015 NW Twenty-second Avenue
Portland, OR 97210
503-413-7673, fax: 503-413-6919

Sleep Disorders Laboratory
Providence Medical Center
4805 NE Glisan Street
Portland, OR 97213
503-215-6552, fax: 503-215-6031

Pacific NW Sleep/Wake Disorders
1849 NW Kearney
Portland, OR 97209
503-228-7293

Salem Hospital Sleep Disorders Center
Salem Hospital
Salem, OR 97309
503-370-5170, fax: 503-375-4722

PENNSYLVANIA

Sleep Disorders Center
Abington Memorial Hospital
Abington, PA 19001
215-576-2226

Sleep Disorders Center
Sacred Heart Hospital
Allentown, PA 18102
610-776-5333

Sleep Disorders Center
Lower Bucks Hospital
Bristol, PA 19007
215-785-9752, fax: 215-785-9068

Penn Center for Sleep Disorders
800 West State Street
Doylestown, PA 18901
215-345-5003, fax: 215-345-5047

Sleep Disorders Center of Lancaster
Lancaster General Hospital
Lancaster, PA 17604
717-290-5910, fax: 717-290-4964

Saint Mary Sleep/Wake Disorder Center
Langhorne-Newton Road
Langhorne, PA 19047
215-741-6744

Sleep Disorders Center
Paoli Memorial Hospital
Paoli, PA 19301
610-645-3400

Penn Center for Sleep Disorders
University of Pennsylvania Medical Center
3400 Spruce Street
Philadelphia, PA 19104
215-662-7772, fax: 215-349-8038

Sleep Disorders Center
Pennsylvania Hospital
Philadelphia, PA 19109
215-829-7079, fax: 215-625-9187

Sleep Disorders Center
Hahnemann School of Medicine
Allegheny University of Health Sciences
3200 Henry Avenue
Philadelphia, PA 19129
215-842-4250, fax: 215-848-3850

Sleep Disorders Center
Thomas Jefferson University
1025 Walnut Street
Philadelphia, PA 19107
215-955-6175, fax: 215-923-8219

Sleep Disorder Center
Temple University Hospital
3401 North Broad Street
Philadelphia, PA 19140
215-707-8163, fax: 215-707-7919

Pittsburgh Sleep Evaluation Laboratory
University of Pittsburgh Medical Center,
Montefiore University Hospital
Pittsburgh, PA 15213
412-692-2880, fax: 412-692-2888

Sleep and Chronobiology Center
Western Psychiatric Institute and Clinic
3811 O'Hara Street
Pittsburgh, PA 15213
412-624-2246, fax: 412-624-2841

Sleep Disorders Center
Community Medical Center
1822 Mulberry Street
Scranton, PA 18510
717-969-8931

Sleep Disorders Center
Crozer-Chester Medical Center
One Medical Center Boulevard
Upland, PA 19013
610-447-2689, fax: 610-447-2918

Sleep Disorders Center
Mercy Hospital
25 Church Street
Wilkes-Barre, PA 18765
717-826-3410, fax: 717-820-6658

Sleep Disorders Center
Lankenau Hospital
Wynnewood, PA 19096
610-645-3400

SOUTH CAROLINA

Roper Sleep/Wake Disorders Center
Roper Hospital
Charleston, SC 29401
803-724-2246

Sleep Disorders Center of South Carolina
Palmetto Baptist Medical Center
Taylor at Marion Streets
Columbia, SC 29220
803-771-5847 or 800-368-1971

Southeast Sleep Disorders Center
200 Fleetwood Drive
Easley, SC 29640
864-855-7200

Sleep Disorders Center
Greenville Memorial Hospital
Greenville, SC 29605
864-455-8916, fax: 864-455-4670

Southeast Regional Sleep Disorders Center
3900 Pelham Road
Greenville, SC 29615
864-627-5337, fax: 864-627-9301

Carolina Sleep Services
1665 Herlong Court
Rock Hill, SC 29732
803-817-1915

Sleep Disorders Center
Spartanburg Regional Medical Center
101 East Wood Street
Spartanburg, SC 29303
864-560-6904, fax: 864-560-7083

SOUTH DAKOTA

Sleep Center
Rapid City Regional Hospital
353 Fairmont Boulevard
Rapid City, SD 57709
605-341-8037

Sleep Disorders Center
Sioux Valley Hospital
Sioux Falls, SD 57117
605-333-6302, fax: 605-333-4402

TENNESSEE

Summit Center for Sleep-Related
    Breathing Disorders
Columbia-Summit Medical Center
5655 Frist Boulevard
Hermitage, TN 37076
615-316-3495, fax: 615-316-3438

Sleep Disorders Laboratory
Regional Hospital of Jackson
Jackson, TN 38303
901-661-2148, fax: 901-661-2441

Sleep Disorders Center
Fort Sanders Regional Medical Center
1901 West Clinch Avenue
Knoxville, TN 37916
423-541-1375, fax: 423-541-1837

Sleep Disorders Center
St. Mary's Medical Center
900 East Oak Hill Avenue
Knoxville, TN 37917
423-545-6746, fax: 423-545-3115

Sleep Disorders Center
Baptist Memorial Hospital
Memphis, TN 38146
901-227-5337, fax: 901-227-5652

Sleep Disorders Center
Methodist Hospitals of Memphis
Memphis, TN 38104
901-726-REST, fax: 901-726-7395

Sleep Disorders Center
Middle Tennessee Medical Center
400 North Highland Avenue
Murfreesboro, TN 37130
615-849-4811, fax: 615-849-4833

Baptist Sleep Center
Baptist Hospital
2000 Church Street
Nashville, TN 37236
615-329-6306, fax: 615-284-4781

Sleep Disorders Center
Centennial Medical Center
2300 Patterson Street
Nashville, TN 37203
615-342-1670

Sleep Disorders Center
St. Thomas Hospital
Nashville, TN 37202
615-222-2068

TEXAS

Sleep Disorders Center
Northwest Texas Hospital
Amarillo, TX 79175
806-354-1954, fax: 806-351-4193

Sleep Disorders Center for Children
Children's Medical Center of Dallas
1935 Motor Street
Dallas, TX 75235
214-640-2793, fax: 214-640-7671

Sleep Medicine Institute
Presbyterian Hospital of Dallas
Dallas, TX 75231
214-345-8563, fax: 214-750-4621

Sleep Disorder Center
Columbia Medical Center East
El Paso, TX 79925
915-595-9246

Sleep Disorders Center
Columbia Medical Center West
1801 North Oregon
El Paso, TX 79902
915-521-1257

Sleep Disorders Center
Providence Memorial Hospital
El Paso, TX 79902
915-577-6152

Sleep Consultants
1521 Cooper Street
Fort Worth, TX 76104
817-332-7433, fax: 817-336-2159

Sleep Disorders Center
Columbia Spring Medical Center
8850 Long Point Road
Houston, TX 77055
713-973-6483, fax: 713-722-3248

Sleep Disorders Center
Baylor College of Medicine and VA
    Medical Center
Houston, TX 77030
713-798-4886 or 713-794-7563

Sleep Disorders Center
Scott and White Clinic
2401 South Thirty-first Street
Temple, TX 76508
817-724-2554

UTAH

Intermountain Sleep Disorders Center
5770 South
Murray, UT 84106
801-269-2015, fax: 801-269-2948

Intermountain Sleep Disorders Center
LDS Hospital
Salt Lake City, UT 84143
801-321-3617, fax: 801-321-5110

Sleep Disorders Center
University Health Sciences Center
50 North Medical Drive
Salt Lake City, UT 84132
801-581-2016, fax: 801-585-3249

VIRGINIA

Fairfax Sleep Disorders Center
3289 Woodburn Road
Annandale, VA 22003
703-876-9870

Virginia-Carolina Sleep Disorders Center
159 Executive Drive
Danville, VA 24541
804-792-2209, fax: 804-799-8037

Sleep Disorders Center
Sentara Norfolk General Hospital
600 Gresham Drive
Norfolk, VA 23507
757-668-3322, fax: 757-668-2628

Sleep Disorders Center
Medical College of Virginia
Richmond, VA 23298
804-828-1490, fax: 804-828-1481

Roanoke Sleep Disorders Center
Carilion Roanoke Community Hospital
Roanoke, VA 24029
540-985-8526, fax: 540-985-4963

Sleep Disorders Center
Virginia Beach General Hospital
Virginia Beach, VA 23454
757-481-8168, fax: 757-496-6337

WASHINGTON

St. Clare Sleep-Related Breathing
  Disorders Clinic
St. Clare Hospital
Lakewood, WA 98499
206-581-6951

Sleep Apnea Lab
Auburn Regional Medical Center
Auburn, WA 98001
253-735-7520

Sleep Disorders Center
Providence St. Peter Hospital
Olympia, WA 98506
360-493-7436, fax: 360-493-4173

Sleep Center
Valley Medical Center
Renton, WA 98055
206-575-3379

Richland Sleep Laboratory
800 Swift Boulevard
Richland, WA 99352
509-946-4632, fax: 509-942-0118

Highline Sleep Disorder Center
Highline Community Hospital
Seattle, WA 98166
206-325-7396

Providence Sleep Disorders Center
1600 East Jefferson
Seattle, WA 98122
206-320-2575, fax: 206-320-3339

Seattle Sleep Disorders Center
Swedish Medical Center/Ballard
Seattle, WA 98107
206-781-6359, fax: 206-781-6196

Sleep Disorders Center
Virginia Mason Hospital
Seattle, WA 98101
206-625-7180, fax: 206-340-2057

Sleep Disorders Center
Sacred Heart Doctors Building
105 West Eighth Avenue
Spokane, WA 99204
509-455-4895, fax: 509-626-4578

WEST VIRGINIA

Sleep Disorders Center
Charleston Area Medical Center
501 Morris Street
Charleston, WV 25325
304-348-7507, fax: 304-348-3373

PM Sleep Medicine
3803 Emerson Avenue
Parkersburg, WV 26104
304-485-5041

WISCONSIN

Sleep Disorders Center
Appleton Medical Center
1818 North Meade Street
Appleton, WI 54911
920-738-6460, fax: 920-831-5000

Sleep Disorders Center
Marshfield Clinic
2655 County Highway I
Chippewa Falls, WI 54729
715-726-4136, fax: 715-726-4173

Sleep Disorders Center
Luther Hospital/Midelfort Clinic
Eau Claire, WI 54702
715-838-3165, fax: 715-838-3845

Sleep Disorders Lab
Bellin Hospital
Green Bay, WI 54305
920-433-7441

Sleep Disorders Center
St. Vincent Hospital
Green Bay, WI 54307
920-431-3041, fax: 920-433-8010

Sleep Disorders Center
Gundersen Clinic
1836 South Avenue

La Crosse, WI 54601
608-782-7300, fax: 608-791-4466

Sleep Disorders Center
University of Wisconsin Hospitals and
    Clinics
Madison, WI 53792
608-263-2387, fax: 608-263-0412

Sleep Disorders Center
St. Mary's Hospital Medical
    Center
Madison, WI 53716
608-258-5010, fax: 608-258-6176

Sleep Disorders Center
Marshfield Clinic
1000 North Oak Avenue
Marshfield, WI 54449
715-387-5397

Milwaukee Regional Sleep Disorders
    Center
Columbia Hospital
2025 East Newport Avenue
Milwaukee, WI 53211
414-961-4650, fax: 414-961-8712

Sleep Disorders Center
St. Luke's Medical Center
Milwaukee, WI 53201
414-649-5288, fax: 414-649-5875

Sleep Disorders Centers in Other Countries

AUSTRALIA

Repatriation General Hospital
Adelaide, South Australia

Sydney Sleep Disorders Centre
Annandale, New South Wales

Sleep Monitoring Unit
Benowa, Queensland

North West Private Hospital Everton Park
Brisbane

Sunnybank Private Hospital Sunnybank
Brisbane

Royal Prince Alfred Hospital
Camperdown 2050

ACT Sleep Therapy Clinic
Deakin, Canberra

Austin and Repatriation Medical Centre
Heidelberg, Victoria

Sleep Disorders Laboratory
Malvern, Victoria

Newcastle Sleep Disorders Centre
Newcastle

Royal Newcastle Hospital
Newcastle, New South Wales

Camperdown Sleep Disorders Center
Newtown, New South Wales

Central West Sleep Disorders Center
Orange, New South Wales

Hornsby Sleep Disorders Centre
Waitara, New South Wales

Satellite Sleep Laboratory
Wentworthville, New South Wales

AUSTRIA

Elizabethinen Hospital
Linz

Pulmonologic Center
Vienna

BELGIUM

University Hospital
Ghent

CANADA

McMaster University Medical Center
Hamilton, Ontario

Credit Valley Hospital Sleep Laboratory
Mississauga, Ontario

Sleep Institute of Ontario
North York, Ontario

Royal Ottawa Hospital
Ottawa, Ontario

Northern Nights Sleep Disorders Centre
Thunder Bay, Ontario

Center for Sleep and Chronobiology
University of Toronto
Toronto, Ontario

Silent Partners Sleep Clinic
Toronto, Ontario

Sleep Disorders Centre of Metropolitan
Toronto
Toronto, Barrie, Brampton, and
Richmond Hill, Ontario

The Wellesley Hospital
Toronto, Ontario

FINLAND

Haaga Center for Neurological Research
and Rehabilitation
Helsinki

GERMANY

Sleep Disorders Center
Bochum

University of Munich
Munchen

Sleep Disorders Center
Regensburg

Sleep Disorder Center of Witten
Witten

GREAT BRITAIN

Scottish National Sleep Centre
Edinburgh, Scotland

HONG KONG

The Chinese University of Hong Kong
Shatin NT

IRELAND

St. Vincent's Hospital
Elm Park, Dublin

ISRAEL

Sorkoa Medical Center
Beer-Seva

Lowenstein Rehabilitation Hospital
Raanana

Tel-Aviv University
Ramat Aviv

Technion Sleep Laboratory
Technion City, Haifa 3200

ITALY

Universita di Roma
Roma

KOREA

Samsung Medical Center
Kangnam Ku
Seoul

LUXEMBOURG

Laboratoire de Sommeil
Centre Hospitalier Luxembourg

THE NETHERLANDS

Sleep Centre Westeinde Hospital
Den Haag

Hospital de Gelderse Vallei
Ede

NEW ZEALAND

Sleep Management Centre
Takapuna
Auckland

Southern Sleep Services
Christchurch

RUSSIA

I. M. Sechenovs Institute of Evolutionary
   Physiology
Sankt-Petersburg

SOUTH AFRICA

Universitas Hospital
Bloemfontein

Groote Schuur Hospital
Cape Town

Entabeni Medical Centre North
Durban

Sleep/Wake Sleep Disorders Centre
Johannesburg

Muelmed Medical Centre
Pretoria

SPAIN

Clinica Quiron Valencia
Valencia

SWEDEN

Avesta Hospital
Avesta

Sahlgren's University Hospital
Göteborg

SWITZERLAND

Sleep Disorders Center
1225 Chene-Bourg

THAILAND

Sleep Disorders Service
Songkhla

UNITED ARAB EMIRATES

Neurology Clinic
Al Ghurair Office Tower
Dubai

URUGUAY

Hospital Britanico
Montevideo

Appendix B

Snoring and Sleep-Related Associations

UNITED STATES AND CANADA

American Academy of Otolaryngology, Head and Neck Surgery
1 Prince Street
Alexandria, VA 22314
703-836-4444, fax: 703-683-5100

American Association of Sleep Services Providers
Ambulatory Services of America
9 North Goodwin Avenue
Elmsford, NY 10526
800-540-4485, fax: 914-345-9073

American Sleep Apnea Association
2025 Pennsylvania Avenue NW
Washington, DC 20006
www.sleepapnea.org

American Sleep Disorders Association
1610 Fourteenth Street NW
Rochester, MN 55901
www.asda.org

Association of Polysomnographic Technologists
P.O. Box 14861
Lenexa, KS 66285
913-541-1991, fax: 913-541-0156

A.W.A.K.E. Network
2025 Pennsylvania Avenue NW
Washington, DC 20006
202-293-3650, fax: 202-293-3656

Better Sleep Council
333 Commerce Street
Alexandria, VA 22314
703-683-8371, fax: 703-683-4503

Canadian Sleep Society
Psychology Department
Queen's University
Kingston, Ontario
K7L 3N6
613-545-2480, fax: 613-545-2499

**Citizens for Reliable and Safe
Highways(CRASH)**
116 New Montgomery Street
San Francisco, CA 94105
800-CRASH12

International Snoring Association
805 West Broadway
Vancouver, British Columbia
V5Z 1K1
888-575-1222, fax: 604-708-1934

International Ventilator Users' Network
4207 Lindell Boulevard
St. Louis, MO 63108
314-534-0475, fax: 314-534-5070

Narcolepsy Network
P.O. Box 42460
Cincinnati, OH 45242
513-891-9936, fax: 513-891-9936
www.websciences.org/narnet

**National Center for Sleep Disorders
Research, National Institutes of
Health**
9000 Rockville Pike
Bethesda, MD 20892
301-496-4000, fax: 301-251-1223

**National Foundation for Sleep and
Related Disorders in Children**
4200 West Peterson Avenue
Chicago, IL 60646
708-971-1086

**National Office of Sleep/Wake
Disorders Canada**
3089 Bathurst Street
Toronto, Ontario M6A 2A4
416-483-9654

National Sleep Foundation
729 Fifteenth Street NW
Washington, DC 20005
202-347-3471, fax: 202-347-3472
www.sleepfoundation.org

Parents Against Tired Truckers
P.O. Box 209
Lisbon Falls, ME 04252
207-353-4572

Restless Legs Syndrome Foundation
4410 Nineteenth Street NW
Rochester, MN 55901
www.rls.org

Sleep Disorders Dental Society
11676 Perry Highway
Wexford, PA 15090
412-935-0836, fax: 412-935-0383

Sleep/Wake Disorders Canada
3089 Bathurst Street
Toronto, Ontario M6A 2A4
416-787-5374

INTERNATIONAL

Australasian Sleep Association
Department of Respiratory Medicine
Westmead Hospital
Westmead, New South Wales 2145
Australia

Belgian Association for the Study of Sleep
Sleep/Wake Disorders Center
University Hospital of Antwerp
Wilrijkstraat 10
B-2650 Edegem
Belgium

British Sleep Society
P.O. Box 21
Lisburn, Coantrim BT282SF
Northern Ireland

British Snoring and Sleep Apnea Association
The Steps, How Lane
Chipstead, Surrey CR53LT
England

European Sleep Research Society
21 Rue Becquerel
Strasbourg 67087
France

Finnish Sleep Research Society
Helsinki University Hospital
Department of Neurology
Haartmaninkatu 4
Fin-00290 Helsinki
Finland

Hong Kong Society of Sleep Medicine
Haven of Hope Hospital
PO Lam Road South
Tseung Kwan O
Hong Kong

Insomnia and Snoring Cure Group
Puncheston
Dyfed SA625RN
Wales

Japanese Society of Sleep Research
Department of Psychiatry
Kitasako University School of Medicine
211 Asamizodai
Sagamihara, Kanagawa 228
Japan

Latin American Sleep Society
Departamento Biologica de la Reproduccion
Universidad Autonoma
Metropolitana Iztapalapa
Avenida Purisima y Iztapalapa
Apartado Postal 55535
Mexico City 09340
Mexico

Netherlands Association for Sleep Apnea Patients
DeNye Oanliz 25
9084 An Goutum
The Netherlands

Sleep Group of the French Pneumology Society
Hospital de Haute Pierre
Service Pneumologie
1 Avenue Moliere
Strasbourg 67098
France

Sleep Society of South Africa
P.O. Box 5331
Rivonia 2128
Republic of South Africa

Swedish Sleep Disorder Association
Neurofys Department
Sodersjukhuset
5-11883 Stockholm
Sweden

World Federation of Sleep Research Societies
Thomas-Muentzer-Strasse 22
99084 Erfurt, Germany
e-mail: sleep.congress@t-online.de

Index

About the Authors

Victor Hoffstein, Ph.D., M.D.

Dr. Victor Hoffstein is probably one of the most definitive experts on snoring in the world today. He is a specialist in respiratory diseases and is currently professor of medicine at the University of Toronto Medical School, head of the Respiratory Division at St. Michael's Hospital in Toronto, and member of the medical staff at both the Toronto General Hospital and the Center for Sleep and Chronobiology at the University of Toronto. He studied physics at the Polytechnic Institute of Brooklyn and the University of Grenoble in France, studied medicine at the University of Miami and the University of Toronto, and served a research fellowship in respiratory physiology at Harvard University. He is a past member of the editorial board of the *American Journal of Respiratory and Critical Care Medicine* and has reviewed scientific papers for more than a dozen other journals. His research interests include upper airway physiology and sleep-disordered breathing, such as snoring and sleep apnea. He has published more than 150 scientific papers, lectured frequently around the world, and appeared on many radio and TV shows.

Shirley Linde, M.S., Ph.D.

Dr. Shirley Linde is a best-selling author whose books have been translated into many languages. She has written on science and travel for major magazines, made many appearances on radio and television, and is the author of thirty-five books, including several best-sellers. Some of the books she has authored or coauthored are *No More Sleepless Nights, Dr. Atkins' Superenergy Diet, The Whole Health Catalogue, The Charleston Program, The Insiders' Guide to the World's Most Exciting Cruises,* and *The World's Most Intimate Cruises,* just published. Former director of public relations at Northwestern University Medical and Dental Schools in Chicago, she has been on the executive boards of both the National Association of Science Writers and the American Medical Writers Association, and has served as public relations consultant to hospitals, universities, medical associations, government agencies, and corporations. She has received several outstanding service awards in communications, and is listed in *Who's Who in America, The World Who's Who of Women, Who's Who of Contemporary Authors,* and *Foremost Women of the Twentieth Century.* When not traveling, she lives on the water near St. Petersburg, Florida.